PRAISE FOR

It Hurts

"I was introduced to Kern Olson over a decade ago by Marvin Rosenfeld, the founder of the teaching journal, *Practical Pain Management*. He shockingly said, 'This man is the one person who really knows and understands the gravity of pain and its treatment.' Quite a statement, but I came to believe it. Long before about anyone else, Kern waded into the interface between mind-body-spirit.

"Most psychologists are stymied by the patient who complains of a physiologic symptom such as headache or spine pain, since these complaints are not purely behavioral. But not Kern. His early work in the rural West gained him an interest in headaches. Later, in the 1980s, he became a psychologist in the University of Oregon Anesthesiology Department. There he began to identify candidates with severe pain who had the psychologic underpinning to benefit from purely medical interventions such as implanted stimulators and intrathecal pumps. Among insiders, this work gained him the appropriate title of 'America's First Real Pain Psychologist.'

"It's now been over a decade that Kern Olson has been my confidant and companion in publishing articles in *Practical Pain Management*. To me, aside from his expert writing ability and knowledge of contemporary pain problems, he has an exquisite grasp on the history of pain. As you read this book you will quickly realize that Kern approaches all subjects from a historical or origin-forward approach. To me, it is this quality that separates this book from all other pain books on the shelf.

"In summary, the serious pain practitioner and educator will not only enjoy a pleasant and informative read on a wide range of subjects, but will come to believe that something has been gained from a master who educates us from the ground up."

–FOREST TENNANT, MD, DrPH
Former Editor in Chief, *Practical Pain Management*

*   *   *

"This work represents a lifetime of experience and Dr. Olson's passion for helping those who must confront not only pain but the potential challenges inherent in some health and compensation systems. I particularly liked the selection of case studies and his accounting of the dual role psychologists can find themselves in of being both a therapist and an advocate for patients.

"It's not every day that you get to crawl inside the head of a psychologist to get a glimpse of how he views chronic pain and the people it affects. This view from the "other side of the couch" however is exactly what the reader receives—insights of relevance to clinicians and patients alike from a pain psychologist who has spent literally thousands of hours working with individuals faced with chronic pain. Dr. Olson has devoted his career to caring for and advocating on behalf of people with pain. His book is rich in antidotes, the basics of multidisciplinary care, and offers clear examples for why affective and cognitive factors need to be addressed in any case involving chronic pain. A true gem in this book is his collection of case studies. Representing hundreds of hours of therapeutic work, these cases provide a sampling of the challenges that face both patients and clinicians focused on managing pain for the long term.

"Chronic pain by definition is long term; and its management is not likely to be completed in 8–10 brief sessions. Dr. Olson leaves the efficient algorithms of managed health protocols behind, and takes the reader on a deep dive into the real world of pain and suffering that gets confronted by the many supportive providers needing to advocate on behalf of their patients.

"Dr. Olson knows both sides of the doctor-patient relationship. Being an individual with pain himself, he knows first-hand what suffering can entail. He knows the value of allowing sufficient time for the formation of a trusting doctor-patient relationship, the value of telling one's story of pain, and the wisdom of introducing change when the patient is ready so that alterations in life style have a better chance of enduring. It is clear that Dr. Olson cares deeply for the individuals he has helped and this book represents his desire to pass his insights on to future patients and clinicians so that others may benefit from his experiences and perspective. "

–DAVID A. WILLIAMS, PH.D.
Professor, Anesthesiology, Internal Medicine, Psychiatry & Psychology
Associate Director, Chronic Pain and Fatigue Research Center
Associate Director, Research Development, MICHR, University of Michigan
President, American Pain Society

IT HURTS

A Practical Guide
for
Pain Management

IT HURTS

BY

KERN A. OLSON, PhD

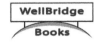

WellBridge Books

WellBridge Books
Portland · OR · USA

ISBN: 978-1-942497-41-7
(eISBN: 978-1-942497-42-4)

Cover Illustration & Design : Jeff Haggen (JeffHagenArt.com)
Technical Editor: Linden Jefferson

Library of Congress Control Number: 2018947517

Publisher's Cataloging-in-Publication

Olson, Kern A., author.
  It hurts: a practical guide for pain management
  / Kern A. Olson.
  p.; cm
  Includes bibliographical references and index.
  LCCN 2018947517
  ISBN 978-1-942497-41-7 (alk. paper)
  ISBN 978-1-942497-42-4 (eBook)

  1. Pain management. 2. Pain-therapy.
    I. Title.

RB127
  616'.0472-dc23

Printed simultaneously in the United States of America, the United Kingdom and Australia.

1   3   5   7   9   10   8   6   4   2

This book is dedicated to my family, past and present:

In memory of my father and mother, Kern and Ruth Olson, whose support and nurturing made me the person that I am today.

To my wife and life partner, Chris, who always gives me honest feedback, and unconditional love and support.

To my beautiful daughter, Catherine Ariane, and my amazing grandson, Tyson River, who is so full of life and loving energy, it humbles me to my core and endlessly delights me.

And most of all to the thousands of my patients who live with pain on a daily basis and who trust me with their stories and their care.

Contents

Preface

WHEN I STARTED THE JOURNEY OF WRITING THIS BOOK, I wanted to make a unique contribution to the pain management literature. I did not want to write another workbook. There are a number of good ones already published. So I thought I would write a type of narrative that would focus on the key factors about pain management that might appeal to the more curious pain patient, and to providers who might not have been exposed to a practical overview of the essential elements in how to work with pain patients. I wanted the reader to experience a conversation with me about pain and how to manage pain, both from a psychological and physical viewpoint. I strongly feel that credible information about pain is the most important tool for health providers and patients alike.

I have been a Clinical Health Psychologist for over 30 years with a specialty in pain management and a sub-specialty in sleep. I became interested in sleep since most of my pain patients reported a sleep issue as a result of their pain. After thiry years of experience, I felt that I had enough experience to share what I have learned as a provider and as a pain patient myself. This book was written for two primary audiences. First, I wanted health providers who work with pain patients to have firsthand "how to" information. Second, I wanted pain patients themselves to be able to access more information and understanding about their own pain management issues.

This book is divided into three main sections. The first four chapters I call the core chapters. These chapters form the philosophical, physiological and historical underpinnings of pain and pain management. The second section contains the specialty chapters that are important to understanding the various aspects of the different types or categories of pain patients. The last section includes seven case studies as an appendix to the book.

I hope after reading this book, the health provider will appreciate the immense complexity of pain management and will become a more effective provider. For the patient who experiences recurrent pain on a daily basis, I would hope the knowledge obtained from this book would provide important tools for your pain management toolbox.

The title for this book, *It Hurts*, comes from our collective childhoods. I would guess the first time you put words to pain, it was something like, "It hurts, Mommy!" This book is designed with that sentiment in mind and I hope the understanding of that hurt will be addressed satisfactorily to the reader. I hope you will learn as much from this book as I have learned in writing it.

Kern A. Olson, PhD
Clinical Health Psychologist
Portland, Oregon

Acknowledgments

A PROJECT OF THIS SCOPE requires support from many individuals. First and foremost, I relied on my wife, Chris, for support and for her skills as a speech-language pathologist. She reviewed and edited every aspect of this project and her input was invaluable. The next phase of editing was performed by my sister-in-law, Linden Jeffers, who works as a professional technical writer. Her work on this project was also essential since she helped polish the manuscript into a professional product.

I would like to thank Brad Simpson, who was kind enough to co-author the chapter on the role of Physical Therapy in Pain Management.

I would also like to thank David Williams, PhD. David is a long-time friend and colleague who is currently at the University of Michigan. David's in depth review of this book was invaluable and his suggestions contributed to the overall quality and improved scholarship.

I am grateful for my friends at *Practical Pain Management* (*PPM*), who have been supportive of my work over the past five years. *PPM* is the largest subscribed pain journal in the world so it gave my work a very wide audience. Specifically, I want to thank Forest Tennant, former Editor in Chief, for his continuing support and valuable feedback, and Nikki Kean, former Managing Editor, and her staff, for their continued support and many kind considerations.

I would also like to thank Denise Williams, Senior Acquisitions Editor of WellBridge Books located in Portland, Oregon. Her comments and thoughtful suggestions gave me the confidence to persevere through the publishing process, which for a new author can be daunting.

Finally, I want to thank my oldest and truest friend, Jeff Hagen, who designed the book cover. Jeff is a well-known and respected artist and author who currently lives in Indianapolis, Indiana. The book cover was inspired by Edvard Munch's *The Scream*. According to Munch, the man portrayed in *The Scream* has lost his soul, and I feel that many patients I have had the privilege to know have also lost their souls. You can visit Jeff at jeffhagenart.com.

Chapter

1 A History of Pain

Study the past if you would define the future.
–Confucius

A Brief Overview from Descartes to the Gate

This chapter covers from the 17th to 20th centuries, from Descartes to the Gate. I have imposed arbitrary parameters and left out many contributors who have played an important role in adding to our understanding of the pain experience. My intent was to include the greatest contributors who appeared to build on one another's work. There were false leads, as in the case of von Frey's work, but his work stimulated new thinking and was significant for that reason. I also included the research that led to Specificity Theory and the response to that model, which is still in use today. The framework for this chapter came largely from Roselyne Rey's book, *The History of Pain*[10] up until the 20th century. The inclusion of Livingston was my responsibility alone, based on my reading and understanding of his work and the influence it had on the Gate Control Theory. From a historical perspective, it is appropriate to end this journey with the 20th century. It is too early to evaluate the contributions that the 21st century will produce.

At the Beginning: René Descartes

We begin our journey of discovery in the 17th century because of one individual, René Descartes (1596–1650), whose research and influence initiated new thinking about pain that has transcended three centuries. Not only did he impact how we think about pain, his contributions to science and medicine was so influential that it is still evident in Western medicine today.

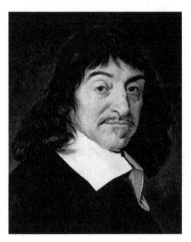

In 1644, his *Principles of Philosophy*[3] was published, in which he discussed pain in phantom limbs. From his observations, he deduced that pain was felt in the brain, not the phantom limb. He introduced his concept of soul: that the soul of pain was located in the pineal gland. He argued that persistent agitation of the nerves from the phantom limb produced sensations as if the phantom limb was still intact.

He believed the pain from the phantom limb was real and not imaginary. Pain was a perception of the soul. Further, he felt that pain was somehow limited to touch and that pain was not a specific sensation, but a more general mode of animal spirits. It is generally believed that Descartes incorporated the notion of the soul to avoid trouble with the Church, being well aware of what had happened to Galileo.

The influence of the Church persisted and was evident up to the 19th century. Traditional Catholic religion maintained that pain is rooted in the passion and death of Christ; that suffering individuals were closer to Christ and that their anguish could be offered up in penance for earthly sins. Church thinking at that time considered pain closely linked to original sin.[10]

In *L' Homme* (1664),[2] which was published 14 years after his death, Descartes presented a model of pain in the form of a boy sticking his foot in a fire. This well-known model has had profound influence on subsequent pain research.

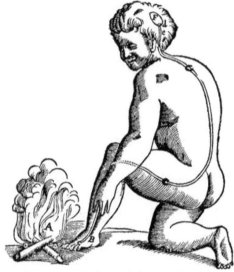

Descartes believed that as the fire came close to the foot, the painful stimulus resulted in the pulling of a delicate thread that ran up the boy's leg to the brain by the shortest route.

Descartes expanded William Harvey's (1628) model of circulation, which embodied the movement of spirits via valves, which acted as little doors opening to let the spirits through and preventing reflux.

Descartes' model of the dualistic nature of pain suggests that pain is primarily a sensory phenomenon that is separated from higher order (neocortical) influences. It is the either/or school of thinking: either pain is physical or it is of psychic origin; they are mutually exclusive.

Descartes' Error

About 20 years ago, I had the opportunity to listen to a lecture in Portland, Oregon, by Antonio Damasio, MD, the M.W. Van Allen Professor of Neurology and Chairman of the Department of Neurology at the University of Iowa, College of Medicine.

He had just published Descartes' Error, in which he stated, "The error is the abysmal separation between body and mind. The suffering that comes from physical pain or emotional upheaval might exist separately from the body."[1]

Damasio stated quite emphatically that medical schools in the U.S. largely ignore human dimensions and concentrate on the physiology and pathology of the body proper. Further, he feels that this neglect stems from a Cartesian dualistic view of humanity that has persisted for three centuries.

The true value of Descartes' research and thinking is that he opened the way to subsequent research on the localization of cerebral functions. He tried to dispel the confusion between pain and sadness. He felt that sadness always followed pain because the soul recognized the weakness of the body and its inability to resist the injuries that afflicted it.[10]

Descartes' work marked a major milestone in pain research and application. He created controversy in the world of pain research, which contributed to more debate and ultimately progress. His research at that time was revolutionary, especially when you consider the level of technology available. His theories were very different and far-reaching as represented by The Boy and Fire. Damasio's critique of Cartesian Dualism is relevant today, especially since there are still many pain providers who feel that pain is only a sensory event.

Damasio's observations were very important, especially considering that the British school of research was influenced by Bacon to advance science through inductive reasoning, and France was influenced by Descartes' reductive mechanistic philosophy. These differences carried on throughout the 18th century.

Progress in the 18th Century

Albrecht von Haller

The 18th century is often referred to as the Age of Enlightenment. A shift in thinking, associated with the decrease of Church influence, was taking place in the secularization of thought and the separation between science and metaphysics. A shift in thinking was also taking place regarding the

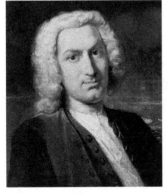

perception and definition of pain.[11] The first major contributor to this shift in thinking was Albrecht von Haller.

He was interested in the reactions of fibers and how to distinguish between the irritability of muscle fiber, which he called the contractibility and excitability of nerve fibers, which he called sensitivity. (In today's vernacular, this would be considered 'hyperesthesia' in extreme forms.)

In von Haller's work, only the nerves are sensitive, while muscle fibers are irritable. Von Haller felt strongly about a strict dichotomy between sensitivity, which was associated with consciousness, and irritability, which was independent of consciousness.

As knowledge and research progressed in the 18th century, a major trend started to develop where research focused on more specific aspects of pain. The specific aspects of pain for von Haller, was the role of muscle fibers and nerves. This is still an area of interest in today's pain research. I would suggest that von Haller's work was the beginning of what we now consider 'myofascial' pain.

Pierre-Jean Cabanis

Toward the second half of the 18th century there was a reaction against von Haller's theory of pain which was led by Pierre-Jean Cabanis (1757–1808).

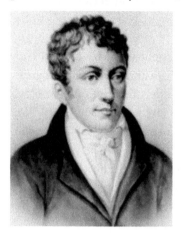

Cabanis's work incorporated a psychophysiological approach to pain, which included the emotional component. For Cabanis, sensitivity could not be defined outside the realm of pleasure and pain, since what affects us can never be indifferent to us.[11] Psychologists and physiologists felt that pleasure and pain always manage to balance each other out. Today we would consider this 'homeostatic' drive, which I believe has profound implications for the pain patient.

Keep in mind that the field of psychology grew out of physiology. This was true in Europe under the influence of Wilhelm Wundt, and in the U.S. under the influence of William James. For Cabanis, pain was useful. It instilled stability, balance, and equilibrium to the nerves and muscular systems. The idea of the usefulness of pain led to the therapeutic techniques of electrical shock and stimulation.

Cabanis also felt that sensations (pain) could be generated spontaneously in the brain and provoke pains that were real. Here he introduces the concept of hypochondria and pain: pain is not a pure physiological reaction to a stimulus, but requires the mental activity of the patient.

It seems to me that Cabanis was either extending Cartesian dualism; pain separate from the physiological perception (dualism) or was inferring that pain was somehow a combination of physiology and psychology.

According to Roselyne Rey, author of the book *The History of Pain*,[10] the work of Cabanis focused on sensitivity as the cornerstone for life, and pain provided the ideal experience to study the relationship between the physical and mental.

Cabanis's questions about the psychophysiological conditions necessary for pain to reach consciousness led him to view the perception of pain as being a complex, chronologically-staged process. During this process, any given sensation at any given time could be absorbed by another sensation. He proposed a competitive model between external and internal feelings, where the weakest sensations were absorbed by the strongest.[11]

Cabanis's research and ideas were a major step forward in how the pain patient was treated. His work led to new techniques, such as using electrical stimulation for the treatment of pain. He introduced the concepts of psychophysiology and the emotional components of pain. These concepts continued to grow well into the 19th century, even though his thinking contradicted von Haller's theories.

Rey observed that there were three different medical philosophies in the 18th century:

- First, there was the mechanical school of thought, those who wanted to return to the notion that the human body functions as a simple machine, which was popular up until the middle of the 18th century.
- Second, there was the vitalist school of thinking, which was more dominant toward the end of the century. They adopted the concept of sensitivity, which included the simultaneous concepts of physiology and psychology.
- Third, the minority school of thought (animism) felt that nature was more passive. It accepted mechanical explanations and considered the soul to be directly responsible for all organic functions. Further, it made pain an important sign in illness as a result of internal strife.[10]

Xavier Bichat

The next major contributor to consider is Xavier Bichat (1771–1802). Bichat's work represented a passage from organic sensitivity to animal sensitivity and the 'threshold concept.' His work on the two nervous systems and their relationship to the understanding of pain was an important contribution. He separately studied the sympathetic and parasympathetic systems, which, in the 18th century, was highly significant. He believed the two systems were very distinct, each having two principal centers, one in the brain and the other in the ganglions. Pain coming from the ganglions was very different from pain coming from the spinal nerves. This distinction agreed with the vital-

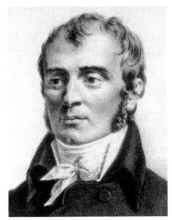

ists, but differed from von Haller. This debate between Bichat and von Haller persisted for over a half century and had major consequences for physiology and the treatment of pain.

Bichat's work complemented the work of Cabanis, which led to a more global psychophysiological approach to pain treatment. This approach also led to the increasing use of opium as a treatment, which was not present in the 17th century.[10]

The work of Cabanis and Bichat represented the beginning of an important trend in pain treatment. They initiated a more holistic approach to pain treatment that is represented today as a multidisciplinary approach to pain treatment.

The 19th Century Advances

Scientific forces that had been building in the 18th century carried over to the 19th century, which saw an increased number of breakthroughs in the understanding of pain mechanisms and therapeutic innovations. The 19th century also saw physiology dominated by experimental research on the structure and function of primary organs which play a role in pain.[11]

Finally, after 40 years at the patients' bedside or in autopsy rooms, physicians began pursuing the study of pain symptoms. Medical texts in the early part of the 19th century started to focus on the links between physical and mental aspects of pain.[11]

The early part of the 19th century also saw the development of clinics, which increased interest in the study of pain. Pain research and thinking at this time remained within the framework of 'specificity theory' advanced by Johannes Müller and Maximilian von Frey. The specificity theory was contrary to their clinical observations and the emergence of endocrinology, which indicated that pain was more complex. In France, the Church again opposed materialism and spiritualism and was concerned that research was reducing the mental aspects of pain to a more physiological/chemical level. According to Rey, this conflict prevented a more complete understanding of pain, and it hardened the positions of each side.[11]

In the middle of the 19th century, there was a debate whether pain could be avoided or accepted fatalistically. This debate was prompted by the role of war, which promoted further progress in the understanding of pain. Many new treatment options were introduced in England, France, and the U.S., including nitrous oxide, the isolation of morphine in Germany, and ether in the U.S.

The number of new developments in knowledge and research was growing. This knowledge was accumulating at such a rapid rate, it created energy for more advances.

Two major contributors were responsible for this rapid accumulation of knowledge, Johannes Müller and Maximilian von Frey.

Johannes Müller

According to Rey, advances in microscopy benefited the work of Johannes Müller (1801–1858) in Germany. He concluded that there were specific energies within the nerve fiber. Further, he concluded that the paths of nerve fibers were rigorously ordered. This research led to his conclusion that there were specific fibers for pain or receptors (neuroreceptors) for painful sensations. This finding was a major step forward in understanding pain transmission. He formulated Müller's *Law of Mechanisms of Sensory Nerves*.

He presented the idea of specialization with respect to the effects of a given stimulus applied to an area restricted to the branches of the nerves found below the point of stimulation. Müller used amputees in his research, since all the primitive fibers were found at the level of the stump and the nerve trunk remained intact. The sensation received by the brain was the same.[11]

Müller then proposed a model where each posterior root ganglion would function like a semi-conductor of the sensation. This model may represent the first step toward the concept of a gate that we will cover later in the findings of the 20th century. He believed that the reaction of a feeling produced by a sensory nerve would occur in the sensory nerves and not the motor nerves. He stated that "the central parts of the sensory nerves that transmit to the brain are capable of feeling independently of the nerve cords or conductors. Sensations are determined appropriate to each sense."[11]

Müller proposed a theory for pain which took into account findings from physiology, historical observations, pathological findings, and integrated psychological dimensions of pain. He believed that pain was not imaginary, that pain could occur without an external stimulus.[11]

His thinking was similar to that of Cabanis, which we discussed earlier. He concluded that pain transmitted from the periphery toward the center traveled through a series of complex relays, which could modify the sensation. This important finding can be traced back to Descartes' models of pain transmission (The Boy and Fire). Müller's model encompassed significant scientific advances largely due to the improvement of the microscope.

Toward the end of the 19th century, research started to focus on receptors that were specific for pain. The advanced microscopes allowed the identification of neural structures, which were very different from one another. Müller felt that these structures served very different functions. This research trend represented another major step toward the Theory of Specificity.[11]

Maximilian von Frey

Maximilian von Frey (1852–1932) elaborated on the work of Müller. However, von Frey's work had very different implications, and led to a more restricted concept of pain.
He was trying to identify particular points in the skin which responded specifically to one of the four cutaneous sensations: touch, heat, cold, and pain. In order to accomplish this task, he invented

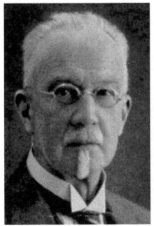

what he called an aesthesiometer, where the stimulus consisted of hair.

The result did not depend on pressure alone, but on location. Further, he felt that pain was perceived when the stimulus went beyond a certain threshold, and this led to his conclusion that pain results from the stimulation of special organs. Von Frey's theory was based on the mechanisms of pain that he felt were dependent on a specific neural apparatus. Today, von Frey's theory has been generally discounted, but his work contributed to the understanding of sensory receptors and the measurement of insensitivities of stimuli and sensory thresholds.[11]

According to Rey, every attempt to establish the notion of specificity at the fiber or receptor level, including transmission, turned out to be insufficient in understanding pain. The methodology of reductionism led to the basic explanation that pain is a simple response to a stimulus.[11]

Also during the middle of the 19th century in Germany, the field of psychology was developed by Wilhelm Wundt, who started the first experimental psychology laboratory in Leipzig in 1859. The Zeitgeist (spirit of the time) in Germany at this time was a focus on measuring reaction times and psychophysics. His research was important to Müller and von Frey's approach to the study of pain.

Bridging the 19th and 20th Centuries

Alfred Goldscheider

Toward the end of the 19th century, and the beginning of the 20th century, the work of Alfred Goldscheider (1858–1935) greatly contributed to the understanding of pain. His research started at the end of the 19th century but was published into the 20th century.

Much of the research of the 19th century carried over to the beginning of the 20th century, with the focus on looking for specific pain points and associations. This focus of research did not generate positive results. The lack of results led Goldscheider to propose a different theory based on three types of research findings.[10]

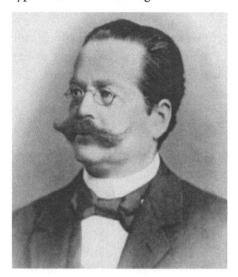

According to Rey:

- The first finding was that the increase of pain upon repeated applications of a stimulus was out of proportion with the intensity of the stimulus. Goldscheider believed this cumulative process acted at the spinal cord and the brain. In my opinion, this finding appears to be the first mention of what is now considered central sensitization.

- Second, he found that when pressure was applied to the skin with the head of a pin, the subject initially felt pressure, then after a short while, the sensation of pain.

- Finally, he found that there were areas devoid of pressure points that turned into pain points.[10]

Goldscheider tried to find an explanation regarding the intensity of the stimulus which brought him back to the theory of 'central summation.' In 1920, he published an collection of his work that started in 1898. He postulated that the difference perceived by tickling, touch, and pain was not due to specific receptors, but due to the bifurcation of the nerve fibers and the routes from the periphery to the center through posterior horns. He felt there would not be specific fibers for pain but special pathways that depended on stimulus intensity. The more frequently a receptor or fiber reacted in a given direction the more the effects of stimuli would tend to take this path.

I believe that his work was a significant step forward and inspired a number of theories in the 20th century, including the Gate Theory.[10] The transition of knowledge from one century to another does not move forward in large steps, but builds momentum, similar to a large wave gaining force as it nears land. The ideas that were produced throughout the 19th century set the stage for major developments in our understanding of pain in the 20th century. The concept that peripheral receptors were structurally diversified and specialized was now accepted, although the existence of specific pain receptors had not yet been discovered.

The 20th Century

According to Rey, at the beginning of the 20th century, research on pain focused on problems of communication, speed, and efficiency. There were two dominant pathways that pain research focused on during the first half of the 20th century.

- First was the temporal aspect of pain mechanisms. This shifted the focus away from specific receptors, transmission pathways, and central organs to time and space factors, conduction rate of nerve impulses, and the study of temporal summation. This shift included studying the connection between mental processes and pain, both intellectual and emotional.

- The second major focus came about with the introduction of Darwin's theory of evolution. It introduced the notion of adaptation in the transmission of sensations and viewed the nervous system as a defense against aggression.[10]

At the beginning of the 20th century, knowledge of pain had reached a new level. The "zeitgeist" within the world of research moved forward now that the influence of the Church was subsiding.

Henry Head

This evolutionary movement in knowledge set the stage for Henry Head (1861–1948). In 1911, he proposed a model indicating the relationship between the cortex and the thalamus

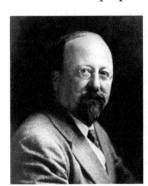

based on his observation of the thalamic syndrome. He felt that thalamic lesions seemed to modify the emotional or affective tone to any perceived sensation. He concluded that the thalamus appeared to influence or amplify sensations transmitted by afferent tracts.

Head determined that the thalamus had three major functions.

- It was the terminus for all afferent sensory pathways which were then redistributed in two directions, first, to the cortex and the body of grey matter in the thalamus, and second that this grey matter represented the center for certain sensations and complemented the sensory cortex.

- The lateral portion of the thalamus served as a receiving station for fibers from the cortex. Head then concluded that the optic thalamus was the center of consciousness.[4]

He believed that the sensation of pain could not be explained with a linear theory of pain. This idea was introduced by Muller in the 19th century, but Head's research gave it more credibility. His model has continued to inform pain research throughout the 20th century. His work emphasized the dynamic connections between various levels which can be observed by the Gate Control Model of Melzack and Wall.

Finally, Head's work should be remembered for its recognition of the role of evolution and that man's evolutionary goal was to ultimately control his emotions and instincts.

Charles Sherrington

The work of Charles Sherrington (1857–1952) was another major contribution to the study of pain in the 20th century. He was a Cambridge neurophysiologist, who received the Nobel Prize for medicine in 1932.

His best known work was the *Integrative Action of the Nervous System*, published in 1908. He transposed the theory of evolution to the level of the neuron and the synapse. He coined the term 'synapse' for the space separating two neurons. Sherrington studied the integration of the nervous system. He focused first on the simple reflex arc, the composite actions resulting from

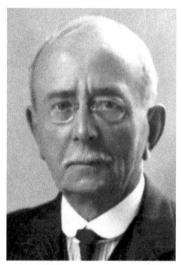

several coordinated reflexes. He studied the simple reflex arc unit's construction, which was the predecessor of the motor unit concepts. Sherrington concluded that the nervous system did operate as a single integrated whole. He earned the Nobel Prize for this work.

The simple reflex was the first step in this coordinated process. He believed that the activity produced by the effector was the appropriate response to the stimulus transmitted by the receptor, which called several neurons into play. "The main function of the receptor is to lower the excitability threshold of the arc for one kind of stimulus and to heighten it for all others."[10, 11]

Sherrington classified stimuli on the basis of their origins into three categories:

1. Proprioceptive receptors—stimuli arising from organs deep in the body, muscles, joints, tendons, and blood vessels.

2. Exteroceptive receptors—found over the entire surface of the body.

3. Interoceptive receptors—includes digestion and absorption known as the visceral sense.[11]

Sherrington's body of work represented a major step forward that moved pain research away from specificity to a more global approach. Further, his work reinforced the role emotion played at the site of the nociceptor.

Edgar Douglas Adrian

Electrophysiology was an important development in the early 20th century. The most significant development was the cathode ray oscillograph. This invention was helpful in understanding that nerve propagation was dependent upon changes in the nerve excitability and conductivity.

Edgar Douglas Adrian (1889–1977), who published the Basis of Sensation in 1928, contributed to these developments.[10] He shared the Nobel Prize in 1932 with Charles Sherrington for work on the function of neurons.

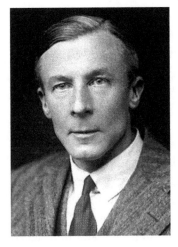

By using the oscillograph, his research focused on how quickly the stimulus generated an electrical current that would result in pain and how long it would last. He concluded that nerve impulses do not travel at the same speed. This concept proved decisive in identifying pain fibers. Adrian concluded that the duration and intensity of a painful stimulus would go through a 'summation' process in order to reach the central nervous system (CNS), and that brief stimuli would not. He also concluded that intensity was dependent on the size of the fiber. This finding was consistent with the All or None law.[10]

Advances in electrophysiology also assisted Thomas Lewis, of London's University College Hospital, in 1942, to conclude that there were two types of fibers responsible for transmitting pain to the CNS, some fast and others slow.[10] The advances in electrophysiology during this period led to the identification of specific pain fibers that is still used today.

As research and thinking progressed through the 20th century, we see a shift away from specificity theory toward a more global approach.

William K. Livingston

In 1989, I helped start the multidisciplinary pain program, which was associated with the Department of Anesthesiology. At that time, I was not aware that the first multidisciplinary pain program was started at the University of Oregon Medical school (later to become OHSU) in the late 1940's under the direction of William K. Livingston (1892–1966). During WWII, he joined the Navy as a surgeon. He was interested in peripheral nerve injuries and soon became head of the Oakland Naval Hospital's Division of Peripheral Nerve Injuries. He published his first book, *The Clinical Aspects of Visceral Neurology,* in 1935, and then Pain Mechanisms in 1943. His third book, *Pain and Suffering,* was started in 1956.[6] In 1966 he passed away before finishing the final manuscript where it was held for safe keeping by the OHSU library. John Liebeskind acquired the manuscript for the *History of Pain Collection* housed at the Louise M. Darling Biomedical Library at UCLA. Howard Fields and the ISAP Press completed the manuscript and it was published by the ISAP Press in 1998.

In 1947, Livingston accepted the position of Chairman of the Department of Surgery at the University of Oregon Medical School. One of his conditions for accepting this position was that he could start a "pain project" in which a team of investigators would conduct research on the physiological and psychological aspects of pain. This project evolved into the first multidisciplinary pain clinic in the U.S. One of the first fellows Livingston hired was a young psychologist by the name of Ron Melzack. His team decided "as our basic assumption the concept that nothing can properly be called pain unless it is consciously perceived as such."[5] With this basic assumption, Livingston opened the aperture further than anyone we have discussed. By then, he considered pain a perception, not a simple sensory event.

By the 1950s, Livingston's thinking had evolved from exploring sensory nerve pathways to a broader interpretation of brain function and its relationship to the perception of pain. "That pain is not always measurable in terms of stimulus intensity. Because we now know that the brain has the

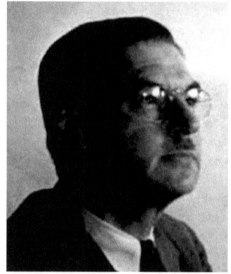

power to suppress the sensory signal before it can ascend to the brain. Further, he states that emotional states can augment the perceptual impact, and that it is a dynamic process that is constantly being tuned to the needs of the individual from moment to moment."[5]

Livingston's work at the University of Oregon Medical School, along with his team, concluded that pain was not mechanistic. His evidence suggested that pain was the direct result of activation of specific sensory receptors at the body periphery, which appeared to be higher up along the conducting pathways or within the CNS. Their evidence showed that the pain and temperature tract in the spinal cord was not the sole route by which pain signals could ascend to perceptual levels, because signals could take many indirect routes. Many of these indirect routes or backdoors allowed signals to bypass any point of interruption on any given tract. Finally, his research indicated that the cerebral cortex was not the true center for pain perception, as responses to noxious stimuli could take other routes in the core of the brain to reach subcortical structures and areas of the cortex outside the somatosensory region. He felt that the brain exerts a downstream influence on all sensory input.[5]

Physiology vs Psychology: Repudiating the Either/Or Dichotomy

In *Pain and Suffering*, Livingston wrote extensively about the role of psychology and pain. In Chapter IV entitled, "The Psychology of Pain," he talked about the difficulty encountered in the search for a satisfactory definition of pain. He felt that any definition of pain could not be considered from either a physiological or a psychological approach. Any consideration of pain by one approach alone or without due regard to the other is incomplete.[5] He was avoiding the old dualistic dichotomy, or what I referred to earlier as the either/or school of thinking.

Livingston strongly believed that pain is a perception; that it is subjective and individual, that it varies in different races of people and that individual susceptibility to pain may vary with changes in emotions and physical equilibrium. Pain can only be evaluated by the individual experiencing it. The human animal is the only one who can analyze his sensations and describe it to someone else.

For Livingston to classify certain types of pain as "psychic" pain is purely arbitrary because all pain is a psychic perception. Further, he states there is a rather widespread tendency to use this term loosely to apply to cases in which there is not an obvious organic origin for the pain.[5]

In my opinion, he is closing the door on the dualistic notion of conversion as proposed by Freud and others throughout the past two centuries. Although, it is interesting to note that in the *DSM I*, it was called conversion, and in the *DSM IV*, it is referred to as somatoform pain disorder. It still implies conversion. I am hopeful that the *DSM V* will finally catch up with current creditable research and eliminate this outdated notion.

The Vicious Cycle of Pain

In Chapter XV of *Pain and Suffering*, Livingston wrote about the vicious circle of pain (causalgia). He states that, "An organic lesion at the periphery involving a sensory nerve may be the source of constant irritation. Further, that afferent impulses from his 'trigger point' eventually creates an abnormal state of activity in the internunical neuron centers of the spinal cord gray matter. This disturbance is then reflected in an abnormal motor response from both the lateral and anterior horns. This muscle spasm, vasomotor changes, and other effects, which the central perturbation of function brings about in the peripheral tissues, may contribute new sources for pain and new reflexes. A vicious cycle of activity is created. If this process is permitted to continue it spreads to new areas and acquires momentum that is increasingly difficult to displace."[5]

Ron Melzack and Patrick Wall

We've set the stage for the next two major contributors: Ron Melzack (1929–) and Patrick Wall (1925–2001).

Fortunately, I had the opportunity to listen to Ron Melzack and Patrick Wall speak on many occasions. Every time was pleasant and stimulating. Unfortunately, Patrick Wall is no longer with us. Ron Melzack is still productive and continues his association with McGill University in Montreal, Canada.

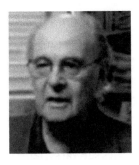 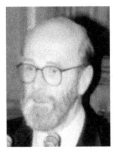

Gate Control Theory

I believe Livingston's influence was the springboard for the next step forward represented by the Gate Control Theory of Pain.

The Gate Control Theory represents a model of pain that is contrary to the dualism school of thinking and the specificity theory of pain, which is still taught in many U.S. medical schools. In 1965, Melzack and Wall proposed the Gate Control Theory of Pain, which suggests that neural mechanisms in the dorsal horn of the spinal cord could act as a gate.

Gate Control Model

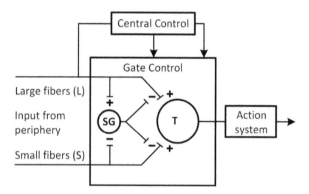

The gate can increase or decrease the flow of nerve impulses from peripheral fibers to the spinal cord cells that project to the brain. They continue by stating that somatic input is therefore subjected to the modulating influence of the gate before it evokes pain perception and response. This theory suggests that large fiber inputs, such as gentle rubbing or vibration, close the gate, while small fiber inputs (evoked by intense stimulation) generally open the gate, which is profoundly influenced by descending controls from the brain. It further proposes that the sensory input is modulated at successive synapses from the spinal cord to the brain. Pain occurs when the number of nerve impulses arriving at these areas exceed a critical level.[8]

Sensory Discriminative and the Motivational/Affective Systems

The output of the T cells (transmission) projects to the Sensory Discriminative system and the Motivational/Affective system. The central control trigger is represented by a line running from the large fiber system to central control processes; these in turn project back to the gate control system and to the Sensory Discriminative and Motivational/Affective systems. All of these systems interact with one another and project to the motor system.[8]

The strength of this model is that it is not linear; that it incorporates several systems in a coordinated fashion and that it includes the emotional aspects of pain as represented by the motivational/affective system. In neuro-anatomical terms, this model opened the aperture to include neocortical influences in addition to limbic influences, and that they communicated with each other in an integrated fashion.

Research that has accumulated since 1965 suggests that the motivational/affective dimension is under the influence of the brainstem reticular formation and the limbic system, which plays an important role in pain. Further, cognitive issues have a profound effect on the pain experience by influencing sensory input in terms of memory, before it activated the discriminative or motivational systems.

Melzack and Wall proposed that the dorsal column pathways act as a feed-forward limb of this loop and that these rapidly-conducting ascending and descending systems can account for the fact that psychological processes play a powerful role in determining the quality and intensity of pain.[9]

In 1989 at the World Congress of Pain, held in Sidney, Australia, the ISAP celebrated the 25th Anniversary of the Gate Control Theory of Pain. At that point, there were over 2,000 published articles engendered by the Gate Control Theory of Pain. Today, the theory continues to thrive and evolve despite considerable controversy. The concept of Gating is stronger than ever. The technology of spinal cord stimulation is based on the Gate Control Theory.

The Motivational Component of Pain

In 1968, Melzack and Casey extended the Gate Control Theory to include the motivational component of pain. In this model, there are three components, usually presented in a Venn diagram of three interlocking circles, with pain at the center, influenced by all three components simultaneously.

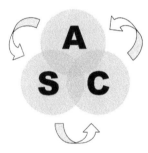

S = Sensory	The sensory component—the discriminative dimension of pain—is influenced primarily by the rapidly conducting spinal systems.
A = Affective	The powerful motivational and unpleasant affect component of pain, which is subserved by activities of the reticular and limbic structures that are influenced primarily by the slow conducting spinal systems.
C = Cognitive	The neocortical or higher CNS processes, such as cognitive evaluation of the input in terms of past experiences that exerts control over both discriminative and motivational systems.

They assumed that all three components interact with one another to provide perceptual information that ultimately influences the motor mechanisms that characterize pain.[7]

2 The Nature of Pain

From the brain alone arise our pleasures, laughter and jests, as well as our sorrows, pain and griefs.
–Hippocrates

The Pain Experience

OUR THINKING REGARDING THE NATURE OF PAIN has shifted over the past four centuries from the linear dualistic thinking of Descartes to the Gate Control Theory of Pain a more global model that includes affective components of pain. The evolution of scientific research has helped us appreciate that the pain experience is more complex and highly multifaceted from the subjective to the specific. We will begin our discussion on the nature of pain with some general assumptions based on our current understanding and then move to more specific considerations.

First, we now know that the pain experience is highly subjective and personal.

Therefore, it is difficult to measure pain using current objective methods. The challenge to the pain provider is that you cannot generalize clinical impressions based on the personal subjective nature of the pain experience. Research in the 19th century focused on measuring the nerve impulses, but this only represented a small part of the global pain experience. The subjectivity of the pain experience is further compounded as the pain impulse moves up the ascending pathways into the brain and reaches consciousness.

Research evidence produced in the 20th century confirmed that the pain experience involves multiple interrelated systems that are highly dynamic. The pain experience can change on a moment's notice, depending on the external demands imposed on our nervous system. Further, the subjectivity of the pain experience confounds today's neuroscientists as they search for more specific intracellular mechanisms to explain the pain experience. After 30 years of experience working with pain patients, it is obvious to me that the pain experience is subjective by nature.

So why is it so difficult to accept the subjective nature of pain? One explanation is that the nature of science has been based on the empirical search for cause and effect relationships and the scientific community is uncomfortable with subjective data. Professionally, I use subjective impressions daily to formulate my clinical impressions and treatment plans.

Second, the individual nature of the pain experience is highly variable.

No two pain patients are the same even though they can be matched on numerous physical social and psychological factors. Because the pain experience is so individual, additional challenges to the pain provider and to the pharmaceutical industry exist. In 1993, I attended the World Congress of Pain in Paris, France. One of the sessions I attended was presented by Patrick Wall, who was discussing some recent MRI results on a specific pain condition. He reported that they found no uniform brain scans across this sample. Twenty years later, I attended another World Congress of Pain in Milan, Italy, where I listened to a very interesting presentation by L. Garcia-Larrea, who presented data from his laboratory. Using functional MRI data, he found uniform responses with a neuropathic pain sample. It appears that we are making progress in research settings that will, hopefully, transfer to the clinical setting.

Third, pain is a perceptual experience, which involves multiple integrated systems that act in a coordinated fashion.

The pain experience as a perceptual process was mentioned throughout the 19th and 20th centuries, culminating with the work of Livingston, Melzack, and Wall.[8,11] When I was a faculty member in the anesthesiology department at Oregon Health & Science University (OHSU), I attempted to impress upon our anesthesia residents that to be effective in working with chronic pain patients you need to treat the patient's perception of their pain. Further, it is important to consider that perception has thresholds, which can be explained by modifications in the periphery after injury or inflammation. According to Marchand, evaluation of these modifications in perceptions often allows us to determine the underlying pathology.[10]

In Chapter 1, I introduced the Melzack and Casey model of pain that was published in 1968. I still use it today to formulate my clinical impressions and treatment plans. Now, I would like to introduce another more contemporary model of pain by John Loeser.[9]

Loeser's Model of Pain

In Loeser's model, nociception is at the center, which is physiological in nature and similar to the sensory component of the Melzack and Casey model.

This model is based on overlying circles, that are actually linear in nature. It starts with a physiological stimulus (nociceptive) that leads to pain (sensory) and results in suffering (affective). Finally, the outer circle represents pain or antalgic behaviors.

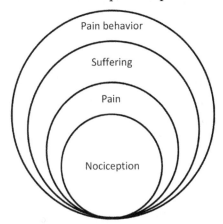

The main difference between the two models is the Melzack and Casey model is circular in nature and all of the components are interdependent. The Loeser model is linear in nature. Accumulating research suggests that our nervous system is highly integrated, interdependent and reciprocal in nature. In addition, the Loeser model infers that the individual components are mutually exclusive which is not consistent with our current understanding of neurophysiology.

Next, we need to consider how we define pain. There are a number of definitions of pain as represented by various pain organizations. The definition that predominates internationally is promulgated by the International Association for the Study of Pain (IASP). In 1979, IASP created a multidisciplinary committee on pain definitions. This led to a standardized definition that was published in the journal, Pain, in 1979, and a supplementary note published in 1982.

"Pain is an unpleasant sensory and emotional experience resulting from actual or potential tissue injury or described in such terms."

The committee also added that pain is a subjective experience. It is associated with our perception of the event and influenced by our past experiences. In my opinion, the IASP definition is based on the work started by Livingston and then continued by Melzack and Wall. It is important to note that this pain definition is not a dualistic, either sensory or emotional experience, but a combination of both, as reflected in the Gate Control Theory of Pain.

We now need to consider how acute pain is differentiated from chronic pain. In other words, what is a normal response to an event such as trauma or surgery as compared to abnormal persistent pain that continues beyond the expected timeframe. This expected timeframe is a hotly debated topic, but generally, it is felt that pain persisting longer than six months (outside the expected timeframe) is considered chronic. There are many in the field, including pain physicians, researchers, and pain psychologists that feel that the passage of time is somewhat of an arbitrary and artificial benchmark. Bonica suggested that chronic pain be defined as pain that persists longer than 1 month beyond the normal healing period or that is associated with a pathological process that causes continuous or recurrent pain over months or years.[2] According to Marchand, the distinction between acute and chronic pain is essential since acute pain plays a protective role and acts as an alarm. Further, it enables us to recognize that there is a problem. Conversely, chronic pain does not play a protective role if it persists long after the triggering event is resolved.[10]

How Pain Works

As we move to more specific considerations regarding the nature of pain, some basics about the nervous system should be reviewed. The history of pain provides valuable background on the evolution of thinking regarding the neurophysiology of pain. To begin this discussion we need to go back to the 20th century and the work of Charles Sherrington, who introduced the term nociception (activity of receptors and nerve fibers caused by potentially harmful stimulation of the body). Today we know that for painful stimulation to reach consciousness, it has to be influenced by mechanisms within the CNS. This influence can increase or decrease the nociceptive stimulus. Further, we need to understand the process of the painful stimulus as it travels from the periphery to the higher centers in the brain.

According to Marchand, "It is well known from nociceptive stimulation to perception, a whole series of endogenous mechanisms (originating from within the organisms) influence our experience of pain. These excitatory and inhibitory mechanisms increase or reduce the nociceptive signal which translates into more or less intense pain."[10] So how does this process begin? To answer this question we need to introduce the term transduction: the process by which the energy of a stimulus is transformed into an electrical response. How does the energy of a stimulus transfer into an electrical response? According to current thinking, the nociceptor has more than one transduction mechanism that could result from direct excitation or through receptor cells. Continuous painful stimulation results in sensitizing the CNS, which contributes to the pain experience.[10]

There are three categories of pain fibers we need to introduce at this time.

- First, there are the larger pain neurons called A-beta: skin fibers responsible for the conduction of non-nociceptive afferents.

- Second are fibers that are smaller and slower called A-delta: these are myelinated skin fibers that play an important role in the localization of noxious stimulation. This suggests they are responsible for the initial pain we feel. In addition, they are also involved in temperature transmission and play a role in the pain we feel from sunburn, where the skin becomes sensitive to touch. This type of pain is a good example of what is called hyperalgesia, an increased response to a stimulus that is normally painful.

- The third category of fibers to consider are smaller, slower, and the most numerous. They are called C fibers. The fibers are small and unmyelinated and are responsible for nociceptive afferents, but because of low conduction speed they pay a role in protecting a painful area. They also play an important role in mechanical, chemical and thermal stimulation. According to Marchand, C fibers are responsible for a secondary pain, which is a later and more diffuse pain, similar to a burn and plays an important role in the intensity of the pain[10]. As I mentioned earlier, they represent 75% of the peripheral nerve fibers and more than 90% of C fibers are nociceptors. Finally, current thinking suggests that C fibers play an important role in the development of chronic pain.

Pathways of Pain Reception and Transmission

Over the course of my pain practice many of my patients have experienced radiating pain. It is especially prevalent in patients who present with severe back or neck injury. This type of pain is quite different from pain generated from the periphery, which infers a different function. Marchand describes a number of characteristics that describe radiating pain. It has different transmission speeds and the precise location does not assume the same importance. Further, radiating pain often develops gradually.[10]. The body reacts instinctively to radiating pain that results in splinting or chronic muscle contraction. We must remember that the body will protect itself when injured by forming a natural splint, which compounds the pain experience by adding another source of pain.

Research that started with Henry Head and has developed over the past 100 years indicates that radiating pain follows certain zones called dermatomes.[5] The path radiating pain follows throughout the different zones will pass through different segments in the spinal cord. The transmission of radiating pain is not well understood at this time. Regardless of this dilemma, Marchand stated, "In all cases the subjective localization of the resulting pain is not representative of the site of pathology."[10]

Dermatomes

A dermatome is a band or region of skin supplied by a single sensory nerve. Sensory nerves carry sensory impulses to the spinal cord—pain, temperature, touch and position sense (proprioception)—from tendons, joints and body surfaces.

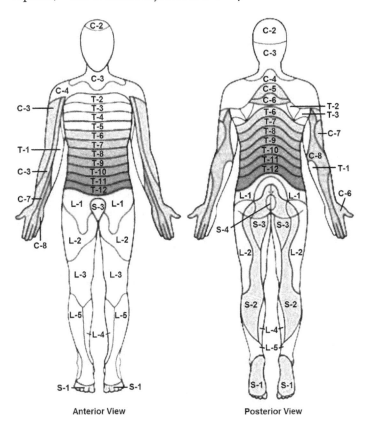

Anterior View   Posterior View

There are two important concepts that need to be introduced in order to fully appreciate the pain experience at the neurophysiological level.

- First, is temporal summation, which results from different speeds between the faster and slower fibers (A-delta and C fibers). According to Marchand, "high frequency repetitive nociceptive afferent stimulation will produce a temporal summation of the nociceptive afferent impulses originating from the slower C fibers. This accumulation of nociceptive activity within the spinal cord is called 'wind up,' which contributes to spinal sensitization."[10] The concept of 'wind up' is important for patients to understand at the clinical level. When I explain 'wind up' to patients I use the example of a light switch to illustrate that pain does not switch on and off, but accumulates or 'winds up.' If the patient understands the concept of 'wind up' they can utilize behavioral techniques to neutralize sympathetic reactivity before it builds or 'winds up.'

- The next important concept to consider is spinal sensitization, which has received considerable attention over the past few years. Spinal sensitization is defined as "an increase in excitability and spontaneous discharge of the dorsal horn neurons of the spinal cord, an expansion of receptor fields and an increase in responses evoked by the stimulation of small caliber fibers (hyperalgesia) and large caliber fibers (allodynia)."[10]

Spatial summation is also important to consider since pain stimuli can cover larger areas on the skin as in the case of severe burns. When you include more nociceptors at the same time it has a multiplying effect on the impulses traveling to the CNS which results in a more intense perception of pain.[10]. Both of these concepts are relevant to the study of fibromyalgia as a chronic pain condition. Recent research has suggested that fibromyalgia patients may have a deficit in the inhibitory system which is not found in other pain conditions.[6]

To continue our understanding of the pain signal, we need to address the transmission of the journey from the periphery to the central nervous system (CNS). This is not an easy concept to explain, because of the variety of receptors and overlap of their receptive fields. In addition, the pain signal is influenced by a number of neuro-chemicals found along the pathways that can stimulate or sensitize the nociceptor. For those of you who are interested in learning more about specific chemical substances, metabolic products and neuromediators, I would recommend Chapter 3 in the *Phenomenon of Pain* by Serge Marchand.[10]

As the pain signal progresses to the dorsal horns (region of the spinal cord where afferent fibers enter the spinal cord) from the periphery, the fibers are separated into two groups: The large fibers, A-beta, enter on the dorsal medial side and the smaller fibers, A-delta and C fibers, enter on the ventrolateral position.[10]

The grey matter, composed of all bodies and the unmyelinated portions of nerve fibers of the spinal cord, is divided into 10 layers or laminae. The A-delta fibers end in laminae I, afferent fibers coming from the deep tissue end in laminae I and V, and C fibers end in I and II. The larger, A-beta fibers end in laminae III or deeper.[10]

Dorsal Horns

At this point in the exploration of pain transmission it becomes very interesting within the workings of the dorsal horns. It is interesting because you have different fibers coming together from different systems that now come in contact with each other. According to Marchand, "The confluence of afferent impulses originating from different systems allows us to better understand the interaction that can exist among systems that seem independent at first. Therefore, muscular pain could be exacerbated by new visceral pain and vice versa."[10] As I explain to my patients, you can experience multiple types of pain, which can act in an additive fashion as the pain experience reaches consciousness.

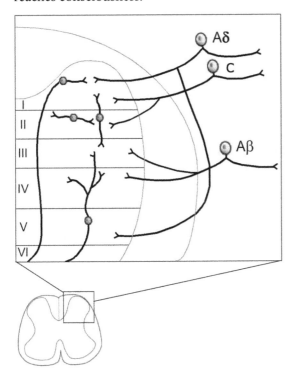

As we move further along in our understanding of pain, we need to discuss what happens to the pain signal once it enters the CNS. Basically, there are three types of neurons that play a specific role.

First, there are projection neurons; neurons with long axons that link it to remote parts of the nervous system, muscles or glands.

Second, there are excitatory interneurons; these are neurons that send the signal from one cell to another and connect signals that are transmitted from the CNS to PNS (Peripheral Nervous System or efferent neurons).

Third, there are inhibitory neurons that prevent activation of the receiving cell.[10]

We can now appreciate the complexity of the pain signal as it enters the CNS. Try to imagine a 3-wire electrical cord, where there are different wires, each with a specific function. Within each of the three major groups of neurons, there are specific neurons with specific functions and some with multiple functions. At this point in our discussion I need to include the role of multireceptive or wide-dynamic neurons. Basically, they gather information provided by primary afferent nociceptors with mechanoreceptors. Wide-dynamic range neurons (WDR) respond in a graduated manner to stimulation.[10] According to Le Bars, these neurons include excitatory and inhibitory areas. Modification of these receptive fields can play an active role in certain pain conditions.[7] A discussion of these specific functions is beyond the scope of this chapter. For those of you interested in a more comprehensive discussion, I would recommend an excellent article by Le Bars.[7]

As the pain signal exits the dorsal horn, the pain pathway becomes more unpredictable based on surgical outcome data. Evidence from ablative procedures that targeted pain-conducting pathways suggests that pain messages travel to the brain by multiple pathways. These findings help explain why sympathetic ablations are not effective in eliminating pain. One pathway that is important to our discussion is the spinoreticulothalamic tract. This pathway is composed of axons that travel from the spinal cord to the brainstem reticular formation before establishing their connection with the thalamus. This tract is divided into the lateral and medial tracts and both are responsible for pain transmission and project to the thalamus.[10] According to Willis, the spinothalamic tract has the necessary qualities for localization and perception. This is relevant for the sensory discriminative component of pain. Further, the spinoreticular tract projects toward the brain stem, thalamus and cortex, which plays a major role in the perception or motivational-affect component.[18] Both of these components have major implications for the Gate Control Theory of Pain.[11]

Spinoreticular Tract

The two above tracts (lateral and medial) project upward to the thalamus, which basically serves as a relay station for almost all sensory information going to and from the forebrain. Keep in mind that the forebrain or frontal cortex is responsible for complex intellectual functions. Prior to the 19th century, pain was thought to be primarily an old brain or limbic phenomenon. Today, we know that the new brain or neocortex, is intrinsically involved in the pain experience primarily due to the thalamus acting as a relay station. The thalamus, therefore, becomes a center for the integration of nociceptive information, which subsequently plays an important role in pain modulation.[10] As we discussed in the chapter on the history of pain, at the beginning of the 20th century with the work of Henry Head, who stated, "pain is a very complex sensory and emotional experience".[15] The development of the MRI, fMRI and PET scans has confirmed that the higher centers in the brain play an important role in the perception of pain. We also know these higher cortical centers contribute valuable influences, such as reasoning and higher order intellectual processing in the perception of pain.

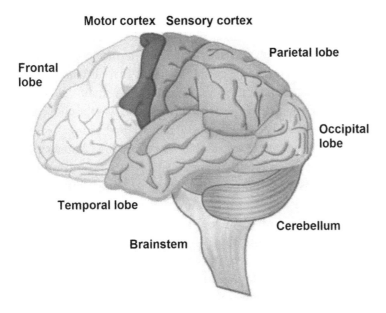

In addition, based on recent evidence we now know there are four cerebral centers that play a role in the pain experience. They are the primary and secondary somatosensory cortex, which processes sensory information (touch, temperature and pain) and is connected to the sensory-discriminative components of pain. Both of these centers are located in the parietal lobe. The third is the anterior cingulate cortex which is located under the temporal lobe. This part of the cortex is part of the old brain or limbic system. Evidence suggests that the anterior cingulate cortex plays an important role in the motivational-affective part of the pain experience. Finally there is the insular cortex, which is located deep within the temporal and frontal lobes. Recent evidence now suggests that this center plays an important role in the affective component of pain.[17] Based on the above findings, we can now fully appreciate Henry Head's comments in the early part of the 20th century. He maintained that the nature of the pain experience is highly complex because of the intricate balance between the sensory and affective components.

The knowledge of the above neurophysiological components now sets the stage for the next step in our journey that began at the periphery and now has arrived at the level of the brain. We now have to consider what happens next to the pain signal, since what goes up, must come down. To begin this discussion, I need to introduce pain modulation that occurs within the body. The Gate Control Theory of Pain influenced our thinking away from linear pain transmission to a model that asserted that the pain signal is modulated once it enters the CNS. Modulation can act either in an excitatory manner, where the pain signal is increased or in an inhibitory fashion, where the pain signal is decreased or absent. It is important to consider that when inhibition is interrupted, it can result in chronic pain.

A number of neurotransmitters are associated with the inhibition system, including serotonin (5-hydroxytryptamine or 5-HT) a monamine neurotransmitter that plays a role in temperature regulation, sensory perception and sleep. The newer class of antidepressant medicines, serotonin reuptake inhibitors (SRIs) are 5-HT based and were initially represented by Prozac. Next is Norepi-nephrine, a neurotransmitter that belongs to the catecholamines. It is produced both in the brain and in the peripheral nervous system (PNS), sympathetic division of the autonomic nervous system (ANS) and produces a variety of behavioral effects including pain inhibition. There is gamma-ami-nobutyric acid or GABA, an amino acid transmitter operating in the brain whose main function is to inhibit neuronal firing. There are a number of non-opiod pain medicines based on the above neu-rotransmitters including antidepressant medicines, such as Effexor, which is a dual acting medicine that blocks the reuptake of both serotonin and norepinephrine and its newer version Cymbalta. The GABA based preparations were originally formulated as anti-seizure medicines, but have now been approved for pain application, the best known is Neurontin.

In addition, we need to discuss the different levels of inhibition that occur within the CNS. According to Marchand, there are spinal mechanisms that are located in higher centers that can be diffuse or local in nature.[10] To further explain spinal modulation, we need to revisit the Gate Control Theory of Pain where Melzack and Wall hypothesized that selective stimulation of the large caliber afferents (A-beta) pain neurons blocks the smaller pain fibers (A-delta and C fibers).[11] Selective stimulation of the afferent non-pain fibers reduces the transmission of pain as it enters the spinal cord, which influences pain only in the dermatome, an area of the skin innervated by sensory fibers from the dorsal root.[10]

On a clinical level over the course of my career, I have evaluated over 5,000 chronic pain patients who were being considered for a spinal cord stimulator (SCS). Spinal cord stimulation is based on the Gate Control Theory of Pain and selective stimulation. My experience and outcome data on the effectiveness of SCS is mixed, which suggests that our current understanding of selective spinal modulation is far from complete.[2, 12, 13, 14, 15] In Chapter 4, The Treatment of Pain, we will discuss spinal cord stimulation in more depth.

Pain is further modulated in an apparent coordinated fashion including a number of areas with-in the brain that involves multiple descending mechanisms. The work of Fields and Basbaum has demonstrated that the rostroventral medulla (toward the front of the lower half of the brainstem) plays an important role in pain modulation.[1, 4]

Further, specific areas involved in descending inhibition include the periaqueductal gray matter (PAG) which is a cluster of neurons located in the pons and nucleus raphe magnus (NRM). Both are contained in the pons located in the hindbrain. The pons is the main structure that receives and transmits information from the forebrain to the spinal cord and PNS. Marchand points out that the two regions contain origins of the descending serotonergic and noradrenergic tracts, which contribute to the inhibition of the pain signal.[10] It is interesting to note that low concentrations of both serotonin and norepinephrine in the cerebrospinal fluid has been associated in fibromyalgia.[16] The above findings reinforce the important usage of antidepressant medicines to improve inhibitory mechanisms.

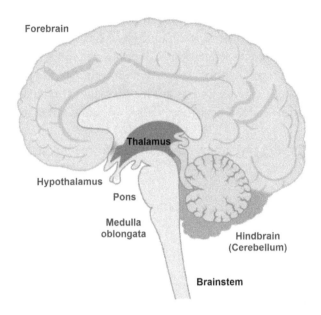

Finally, we need to include the role that the higher centers in the CNS play in pain modulation. Our knowledge has recently improved with the advancement of imaging technology, especially when considering the roles sensory and emotional components play in the higher cortical regions[3]. A number of regions in the higher cortex are involved in pain perception, which relate to the sensory-discriminative component of the Gate Control Theory of Pain. The interaction between higher centers and the limbic (old brain) structures play a role in the motivational-affective component of the Gate Control Theory of Pain. Both of these influences contribute to pain modulation.[10]

Pain research over the last 100 years has emphasized the importance of perception in the pain experience. Marchand has defined perception as the "personal interpretation of the nociceptive (pain) stimulus from an emotional situation and past experiences."[10] I pointed out earlier, the process of pain perception is personal and dependent on the individual's past experiences, cultural influences and psychological status all of which need to be considered when evaluating the patient who presents with chronic pain.

As we conclude this chapter on the nature of pain, we can now appreciate the evolution of thinking from the 17th century to the present time. Our knowledge of the pain experience has moved forward from a simple linear, dualistic model to a more global, intricate model that includes the importance of affective or emotional influences. Advances in neurophysiology and neuroanatomy have improved our knowledge with regard to the role modulation plays in the pain experience. Improvements in imaging have provided valuable information that has resulted in improved care for the pain patient.

In retrospect, the construction of this chapter was a difficult task because the nature of pain is both subjective and complex from a neurophysiological perspective. The challenge was to compose a chapter that included a balance that would appeal to pain patients and pain providers alike. I have attempted to include recent thinking in a meaningful and practical manner. Hopefully, for the pain patient, this chapter provides new information and reassurance that progress has been made. Remember, information is a powerful tool that counteracts superstitious thinking and old stereotypes. My clinical experience over the past 30 years has taught me to never underestimate the patient's quest for knowledge or dismiss their level of curiosity in understanding the pain experience. I believe patients have an inherent drive to try to understand how their bodies work and why they experience chronic pain.

I am also hopeful that all providers who work with pain patients will find the information in this chapter useful in their everyday practice.

I would like to close this chapter by sharing a principle that I have learned to appreciate and use daily in working with patients who experience chronic pain.

Occam's Razor

A logical principle that states a person should not increase beyond what is necessary the number of entities required to explain anything or that the person should not make more assumptions than the minimum needed.

William of Occam 1288–1347

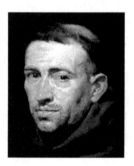

Chapter

3 Pain Assessment

Believe that life is worth living and your belief will help create the fact.
– WILLIAM JAMES, Father of American Psychology

The Psychosocial Assessment of Pain

IN THIS CHAPTER, I DESCRIBE THE ASSESSMENT APPROACHES that I have used over the past 30 years of practice as a pain psychologist, including assessing pain perception and the severity of pain, and evaluating the patient's overall pain experience.

The Patient's Role

The prevalence of pain in the U.S. is staggering. According to the recent survey conducted by the Institute of Medicine, an estimated 111 million people in the U.S. experience recurrent pain. One in four adult Americans report an episode of pain during the last month that persisted more than 24 hours.[18] Data presented from the National Health Survey indicated that within the sample, 15% of adults had experienced migraines or severe headache, 15% experienced neck pain, 27% experienced pain in the lower back, and 4% experienced pain in the jaw.[14]

Pain is the number one reason we go to the doctor (Hing 2006).[9] Ten years ago, according to the Employer Health Care Survey, pain was projected to cost the U.S. economy approximately $100 billion each year. Based on these remarkable statistics, it is imperative for the health care industry to improve and refine assessment approaches so that providers who specialize in pain management can meet the challenge. According to Turk and Melzack, "Pain is not well understood and the severity of the pain may not be adequately managed." They further admit that the central problem in providing appropriate treatment of pain continues to be the inherent subjectivity of the pain experience.[26]

In the chapter on the nature of pain, I mentioned that I use subjective data in forming my clinical impressions and treatment recommendations. Conversely, the provider must remember that the assessment process is a two-way experience, since the patient is also assessing the provider based on subjective impressions. If the patient is unhappy with their provider or treatment, it can influence treatment outcome. The provider and the patient must both keep in mind that pain medicine is not an exact science, but is based on a trial and error, which can be frustrating for both the provider and the patient.

- The first step in the subjective assessment process begins early and plays an important role, since it creates an initial impression that follows the patient throughout the assessment experience. It begins when the patient arrives for the initial appointment. Such factors can include the completeness of the initial paperwork, appearance, and how the patient interacts with the provider's staff. All of these factors can create a subjective impression that becomes part of the patient's permanent medical record.

- Next, under typical circumstances the patient is evaluated by their primary care provider (PCP). The PCP will review initial paperwork and incorporate staff subjective impressions before they actually meet the patient.

After the PCP completes the initial evaluation of the History and Physical (H & P), two possible decisions come into play.

- The first option is that the PCP may decide to treat the patient with pain medicine and conservative treatment, such as a course of physical therapy if indicated.

- The second option may be that the PCP elects to refer the patient to a specialist for further assessment and recommendations. If referring to a specialist, the PCP will forward the initial evaluation that will include subjective impressions. The specialist may elect to perform additional tests before they forward their response back to the PCP. This evaluation may include additional subjective impressions as well as objective findings. The end result is that as the patient's medical record expands, it accumulates subjective impressions that will greatly influence subsequent treatment recommendations.

The Provider's Role

Each provider who participates in the assessment process will have a specific purpose that will form the content of their assessment. In addition, each provider will determine the outcome of initial assessment recommendations. At this point in the process, the assessment and initial recommendations become part of the trial and error treatment journey. The patient should be advised that the provider is charting the course of this journey with some of the following goals:

- formulating a differential diagnosis
- response to a treatment
- understanding the nature of the patient's pain
- the impact of the pain on the patient's life
- the assessment of physical strengths and weaknesses

The provider must be sensitive to the physical and emotional demands placed on the patient by extended assessments.

The Measurement of Pain

The measurement of pain presents a number of challenges to the pain provider. The patient is the only source who can provide information regarding the intensity of their pain. Patients are asked throughout the assessment process to rate their pain is some form of analog scale from 0–10, from no pain to the worst pain they can imagine.

There are a number of concerns with this approach, especially if the provider believes that the patient's rating is a true reflection of the sensory aspect of the total pain experience.

A number of issues arise depending on how you use this information. If you ask the patient to recall their pain level over the past week, as an indication of pain intensity, the unreliable nature of memory becomes evident. A study that examined this issue found that patients will consistently underestimate or overestimate when asked to recall pain levels.[23] When relying on a single measure of pain intensity, the provider is omitting valuable data since pain represents a complex subjective experience. Yet in reality, the patient's rating is usually the only measure that is used in the clinical setting.

Projective Measures

In my practice, I use the patient's rating as a projective measure of psychosocial distress and not a sole measure of sensory perception. I will address this issue from a number of perspectives. The old adage that you cannot tell a book by its cover is relevant to this issue.

There are many providers who feel that the only approach to identify the true nature of pain is to demonstrate physical or chemical pathology. Disability claims, including Social Security rely exclusively on physical findings, imaging and laboratory results in determining acceptance or rejection of claims. The reasoning behind this approach is based on the faulty assumption that physical findings are directly related to the pain experience. Unfortunately, biomedical research has not been able to confirm that the existence of physical pathology and pain are directly related. In fact, a number of studies have found that significant pathology can exist in individuals who report little or no pain and conversely, studies have found significant levels of pain with little or no physical pathology.[2, 4, 10] Turk and Melzack state that "The association between physical abnormalities and patient's reports of pain is often ambiguous or weak. In addition, physical pathology has been reported not to be predictive of disability."[26]

There are still many pain providers who feel that if pain is not associated with physical pathology, then by simple deduction, pain must be psychogenic in origin. As I have pointed out previously, there is no creditable empirical research to support this position. For a more thorough discussion of this topic, I would refer the reader to Chapter 20 of the *Handbook of Pain Assessment,* by Sullivan & Braden.[26]

Assessment Approaches and Techniques

Before I introduce specific assessment approaches and techniques, an important caveat should be interjected. Most of what we know today about the chronic pain experience is based on a very small and select sample of the overall pain population. Our current knowledge base is primarily derived from patients who have been referred to specialized pain programs and not the general population of patients who experience chronic pain.[27]

With this caution in mind, I will attempt to focus on practical assessment approaches that are relevant in today's clinical setting. I would now like to introduce my personal approach to assessment that has evolved over 25 years of practice as a pain psychologist. Further, as I mentioned above, only a small select sample of pain patients will undergo a comprehensive psychosocial assessment. The role of a pain psychologist is very limited due to a number of factors:

- There are very few psychologists who specialize in pain, growing insurance limitations, and patients' reluctance to agree to a comprehensive psychosocial evaluation.
- The majority of pain psychologists are usually employed by comprehensive pain management programs, which are usually located in metropolitan areas.

When I was recruited by OHSU in 1989 to help form a multidisciplinary pain program, there were only two pain psychologist in the entire Portland area. Today, the numbers are improving, but many pain patients, especially in rural areas, will never undergo a comprehensive psychosocial evaluation.

The IMPACT Template

Since no universally accepted template exists to guide a clinical pain assessment, I suggest the Initiative on Methods and Measurement and Pain Assessment in Clinical Trials (IMPACT) be used as a guideline. Even though IMPACT was proposed for research in clinical trials, I feel it has relevance for the general clinical setting.

By 2012, eight consensus recommendations have been published. For a more in-depth review, I refer the reader to: www.impact.org. The four domains and measures recommended by the IMPACT study are the following:

- Pain Intensity
  - 0–10 Numerical Rating Scale
- Physical Functioning
  - Multidimensional Pain Inventory
  - Brief Pain Inventory Interference Scale
- Emotional Functioning
  - Beck Depression Inventory
  - Profile of Mood States
  - Total Mood Disturbance — Specific subscales
- Global Rating of Improvement
  - Patient Global Impression of Change.[5]

Behavioral Analysis of Pain (BAP)

In 1989, I attended a week-long intensive workshop conducted by Wilbur "Bill" Fordyce. Bill Fordyce was a pioneer pain psychologist who helped found the pain management program at the University of Washington. He introduced the term "pain behavior" from an operant theory perspective. Operant theory proposes that pain behaviors are controlled by consequences, which formed the treatment approach at the U of W pain program.[7] During the assessment process, I will introduce a model of pain behavior that can be traced back to B.F. Skinner. Skinner was one of the early pioneers in operant theory.[28] Skinner called his model the ABCs of behavior.

This model is consistent with understanding the nature of pain behavior.

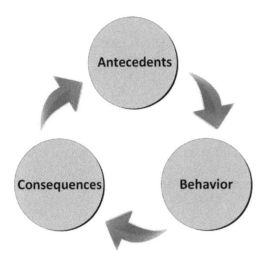

- A represents the antecedent or trigger, which can be an observable situation, such as stress, or a more internal cognitive thought.

- B represents the pain behavior, which can be physical or verbal, such as a groan.

- C is the consequence of B, which could be a negative thought or an observable behavior such as lying down.

Skinner originally presented this model in the form of a circle. This model can apply to pain behavior since pain behaviors can be reciprocal. In other words, a consequence can act as a trigger that sets up another ABC sequence. Once the patient becomes familiar with this approach, I will ask the patient to diagram an ABC sequence from their perspective. This experience is valuable for me as a provider in assessing pain behaviors under operant control and for the patient, since they are now an integral participant in the assessment process.

For me the most important aspect of the Fordyce workshop was how to use his Behavioral Analysis of Pain (BAP). To my knowledge, he never published the BAP so I will summarize it for the reader. It still forms the basis for my initial interview and evaluation.

The main purpose of a psychological evaluation is to determine if pain/suffering behaviors appear to be controlled by social or emotional contingencies or by stimulus control as a consequence of superstitious learning. He felt strongly that the spouse or significant other should also be interviewed. I use the BAP to complement the ABC model, since I am looking for associations between pain behaviors and environmental cues (triggers) and consequences.

Fordyce further recommends the BAP should be complemented by a medical evaluation, a complete pre/post-morbid history and psychometric testing when indicated. There are 19 questions included in the full BAP.

The following is a summary of the 19 behaviors assessed:

1. Describe the pattern or trend of your pain over the course of a day.
2. When is bedtime for you?

3. Once in bed how long does it take to fall asleep?
4. After you are asleep how often do you awake due to pain or other circumstances?
5. When you awake what do you do?
6. When do you get up?
7. How often do you nap?
8. What makes your pain worse?
9. What eases or relieves your pain?
10. What does your pain keep you from doing?
11. How does your spouse or significant other react to your pain? How does it restrict their activities?
12. What is the effect of stress on your pain?
13. What is the effect of deep relaxation on your pain?
14. What is the effect or influence of your pain on sexual activity?
15. How can others around you tell when your pain is bad?
16. How do they react when your pain is bad?
17. Over the past six months what has been the trend of your pain?
18. Looking down the road what do you expect will happen to your pain problem?
19. Given all the information you have, what is your best estimate to why you have pain, or what is wrong with your body?

If a sleep problem exists, I supplement the BAP with a sleep log that the patient fills out over the course of a week.[21] For more information, see The Relationship Between Pain and Sleep in Chapter 5.

McGill Pain Questionnaire (MPQ)

The first psychometric test that I am going to review is the McGill Pain Questionnaire (MPQ), which is based on the Melzack & Casey Model of Pain.

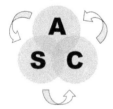

The initial research was conducted by Melzack and Torgerson in 1971 to assess the three major components of the pain experience: sensory-discrimination, motivational-affective and cognitive-evaluative.[16, 17] The MPQ is based on 102 descriptive adjectives that describe different aspects of the pain experience. These 102 adjectives are categorized into three major classes: 1) sensory, 2) affective and 3) evaluative, and 16 subclasses. The MPQ further attempted to determine pain intensities implied by the adjectives within each subclass. Based on a number of studies the MPQ appears to be valid, reliable, consistent, useful, and does not take long to complete.[15] Since its introduction in

1975 the MPQ has been used in more than 500 research studies and has been translated into more than 18 languages.[26]

It is now accepted that the pain experience is a multidimensional phenomenon that requires assessing psychosocial factors that influence the sensory aspect of pain. Over the past 20 years psychosocial assessment has witnessed the introduction of a wide variety of psychometric instruments. It is beyond the scope of this chapter to review every psychometric test on the market today. Therefore, I will focus on instruments that have stood the test of time and more recent tests that show promise and fill a new recognized aspect of the pain experience.

Sickness Impact Profile (SIP)

To assess a broad comprehensive health inventory, I still recommend the Sickness Impact Profile (SIP). I included this test in my original battery and still feel it has value for pain and assessing psychosocial aspects in a general medical population. The most recent version appeared in 1981 and according to the authors it was developed to measure the impact of disease on both physical and emotional functioning.[1] It is a straightforward instrument composed of 136 yes/no questions. The main scales assess ambulation, mobility, body care, movement, social interaction, alertness, behavior, emotional behavior and communication. It also includes independent scales for sleep, rest, eating, work management, recreation and past times. Published psychometric data suggests good reliability and validity.

Multidimensional Pain Inventory (MPI)

One other general psychometric test that I recommend is the West Haven-Yale Multidimensional Pain Inventory (MPI).[12] This instrument is well respected and widely used with a focus on cognitive-behavioral aspects of chronic pain. The 52-item, 12-scale questionnaire is divided into three parts.

Section 1 contains 5 scales:

1. Perceived Interference of Pain in Vocational, Social/Recreational, Family, Marital/Couple Functioning
2. Support from Significant Others
3. Pain Severity
4. Life Control with Activities of Daily Living
5. Affective Distress

Section 2 assesses patients' perceptions of others to their pain. Further scales measure negative, solicitous, and distracting responses.

Section 3 assesses patients' participation in four types of daily activities: household chores, outdoor work, activities away from home, and social activities.

Numerous studies confirm that the MPI is psychometrically sound and that it provides comprehensive information that is useful in the clinical setting.

Cognitive Behavior Therapy (CBT)

Cognitive Behavior Therapy (CBT) as a psychological pain treatment has become the therapy of choice. The role of CBT evolved out of a strong history of behavior therapy that recognized that cognition or thinking was an important component of behavior change. In addition, CBT has gained further acceptance because of a growing empirical research base supporting the strength of this approach.[19]

An important component of the CBT approach is the assessment of the patient's beliefs about pain. Maladaptive beliefs are now recognized as a major risk factor in poor response to treatment outcome.[3]

There are a number of beliefs assessment instruments available, but one that stands out is the Survey of Pain Attitudes (SOPA). The initial version was published in 1987.[11] It has 24 items designed to assess five dimensions of pain beliefs:

1. Pain Control
2. Pain-Related Disability
3. Medical Cures for Pain
4. Solicitude from Others
5. Medication for Pain.

An additional dimension, emotionality, was added in 1989.[11] The SOPA has undergone three major revisions and is now available in two short versions. Research on the SOPA has consistently demonstrated strong psychometric support.

Coping with Pain

An additional component of cognitive pain assessment is how the patient copes with pain. Coping with pain is an integral aspect of Cognitive Behavior Therapy. Lazarus and Folkman, in 1984 defined coping as "constantly changing cognitive and behavioral efforts to manage specific external and/or internal demands that are appraised as taxing or exceeding the resources of the person".[13]

This definition implies that coping is a fluid process that can changed depending upon demands over time. Individual differences can influence coping by beliefs, personality, biology, and social roles. It is important to recognize how the patient appraises pain, since it can greatly influence how they cope with pain: Is the pain killing me or is it troublesome?

Coping Strategies Questionnaire (CSQ)

The one established test that stands out in assessing coping is the Coping Strategies Questionnaire (CSQ).[22] The CSQ was designed to assess specific coping styles. It designates six cognitive and one behavioral coping strategy.

Cognitive coping scales include:
1. Diverting Attention
2. Reinterpreting Pain Sensations
3. Coping Self-Statements

4. Ignoring Pain Sensations
5. Praying or Hoping
6. Catastrophizing.

The behavioral subscale is: Increasing Activity.

In addition, there are two self-efficacy questions assessing perceived control over pain and ability to decrease pain. Overall, the CSQ is widely used, demonstrates research support, and is appropriate in the clinical setting.

One subconstruct of coping that has gained increasing attention since the CSQ was published in 1983 is catastrophizing. Catastrophizing was included in the original CSQ, which focused on a style of reacting to a stressor, including pain. From a pain perspective, catastrophizing has been defined as "an exaggerated negative orientation toward pain stimuli and pain experience.[24] I have, for many years, thought that catastrophizing was a major risk factor. This has only recently gained wider-spread recognition. I refer to catastrophizing as the "Chicken Little Factor". When a patient rates their pain as a 15 on a 0–10 scale, I suspect they are catastrophizing or symptom magnifying. I have also noticed over the years that the patient who catastrophizes will usually score high on Scale 3 of the Minnesota Multiphasic Personality Inventory (MMPI) and Group 6 on the MPQ.

Before I move on to the next section, I would like to point out that I have omitted many psychometric tests that rely on self-reporting. To discuss all the tests that are available today is outside the parameters of this book. For those of you interested in this topic I would highly recommend Turk and Melzack's book on Pain Assessment.[20]

Psychophysiological Techniques

The next section will shift assessment focus to psychophysiological techniques, which should not be considered in lieu of a psychosocial assessment, but should be considered a complementary area of assessment.

My interest in psychophysiology goes back to my undergraduate days when I had a double major in Psychology and Physiology. That early interest led me to using biofeedback, which opened the door to local physicians referring headache patients to me. This was my entry point into the world of pain management, which motivated me to attend the San Francisco Biofeedback Institute and spend a summer with Johann Stoyva, a pioneer in the use of biofeedback with headache.

Sympathetic Nervous System (SNS)

The role of the sympathetic nervous system (SNS) in pain experience has been well documented. In addition, there are many prominent researchers who feel pain is mediated by the SNS. If this assumption is correct, then the psychophysiological assessment of the SNS becomes an important component in the overall assessment of the pain experience. Therefore, I will focus on psychophysiological modalities that can be practically used in the clinical setting and provide important information that complements the overall assessment of the pain patient.

- The first modality mentioned is the surface electromyograph (EMG). It is well accepted that elevated levels of muscle tension plays a critical role in many pain syndromes including headache, temporomandibular joint (TMJ) and low back pain. Flor and Turk reviewed 60 studies using EMG on headache, TMJ and back pain. Their analysis found the results inconsistent.[6] There are numerous possibilities to account for this conclusion including equipment variability and reliability. One study found lower than normal EMG resting baseline levels in fibromyalgia patients.[25] What I have learned from my experience with EMG is that the provider needs to measure resting baseline levels, then introduce a stressor and then assess the patient's muscle reaction and how it influenced their pain. The provider should not be surprised at the wide variability across patients with the same pain presentation.

- The next modality that deserves mention is skin temperature, since it is a valid indication of sympathetic reactivity. In addition, skin temperature/vasoconstriction is associated with stress. This finding has special relevance to patients who experience circulation problems such as Raynaud's Disease. A number of studies have indicated that patients with Raynaud's vasoconstrict more to stress as compared to non-Raynaud's individuals.[8]

- On a practical clinical level, when I introduce myself to a patient, I always pay attention to the patient's hand temperature. If it is cold, I will attach a skin thermistor and monitor skin temperatures throughout the initial interview. This data then becomes part of the evaluation and subsequent treatment recommendations. The practical utility of skin temperature feedback is that the patient can leave the thermistor on as they go about their day. This has two purposes for me in the clinical setting. The first is that it builds awareness of the mind/body connection. Secondly, I will use the skin temperature readings in association with the patient's pain levels. This feedback helps me determine how reactive the patient is outside the office environment.

- The third psychophysiological modality is the electrodermal response (EDR) or, in the old parlance, galvanic skin response (GSR). Skin conductance has been shown to be a good measure of general arousal or sympathetic reactivity. In certain pain syndromes, such as complex regional pain syndrome, phantom limb pain, autonomic arousal, general arousal or sympathetic reactivity appear to play a central role. The research on skin conductance appears to be mixed, which again reinforces the fact that each patient needs to be assessed individually. Then it can be determined if this modality is associated with the patient's pain levels. EDR is relatively easy to use in the clinical setting and does not require expensive instrumentation. Further, as compared to skin temperature feedback, EDR is quicker in terms of reaction time, but in my experience with both modalities, EDR will exhibit more variability.

Summary

In this chapter I left out many psychophysiological modalities, such as blood flow, which is redundant to skin temperature, EEG feedback, heart rate, blood pressure, pupillometry, and respiration. These omitted modalities are now considered to be more appropriate in the research setting and not as practical in the clinical environment because of time restrictions and insurance limitations. The featured modalities of EMG, skin temperature and EDR do not require extensive instrumentation, are relatively quick and easy to administer in the clinical setting, and most importantly can provide valuable information regarding the patient's level of sympathetic reactivity in relation to their pain levels.

To conclude, I would like to point out that a comprehensive psychosocial evaluation needs to include assessment of the patient's mood, fears, expectancies, coping ability, close supportive relationships, and the impact of pain on the patient's life. All of these components complement the physical examination so that the whole patient can be evaluated and treated in the best fashion available. As I mentioned earlier, there is no universally accepted template for a complete evaluation, so the patient can expect to encounter a wide variety of approaches.

A number of factors can contribute to this variability including, the nature of the setting, the experience level of the provider conducting the evaluation, the purpose of the evaluation, whether or not the patient is being considered for implantable pain technology, resources available, including financial considerations and support personnel.

My goal for this chapter was to provide creditable information for the patient who experiences pain, so that they can be more informed as a consumer. I am also hopeful the provider will appreciate the value of a comprehensive psychosocial, physiological, and behavioral evaluation that reinforces the view that chronic pain is a complex phenomenon.

In the next chapter on the treatment of pain, I will describe additional assessments, such as assessment of chemical dependency and specialized assessments.

4 The Treatment of Pain

The stronger person is not the one making the most noise but the one who can quietly direct the conversation toward defining and solving problems.
–Aaron T. Beck, MD (1921–) Founder of Cognitive Behavioral Therapy

A Multidisciplinary Approach to Chronic Pain

I HAVE A DEEPLY-HELD CONVICTION that the best treatment of chronic pain is a multidisciplinary approach, not an either/or option. Chronic pain should not be just treated medically and then if that fails, refer the patient to psychological treatment. This is the worst-case scenario for the patient and the pain psychologist since the patient will interpret that "my pain must be all in my head."

This conviction evolved over my 25 years of practice. I have been fortunate throughout my career to work with excellent surgeons and pain management physicians who have shared with me what is appropriate in terms of medical management for chronic pain. I feel that interventional procedures can be appropriate if the patient is carefully screened by a pain psychologist and by the physician who is going to perform the elective procedure.

Twenty years ago I was invited to join a small, select group of spine surgeons to form a website. At that time the World Wide Web was just beginning and we had no idea where this endeavor would go. Today *Spine Universe* has over 200 distinguished faculty members and receives over 2 million hits per/week. I am still a contributing member of that faculty and I learn of new techniques and developments on a continuing basis from periodic updates and feedback.

My experience as a pain psychologist at the OHSU Multidisciplinary Pain Program taught me to appreciate how various disciplines can work together to provide optimal pain treatment. While at OHSU, I was appointed to sit on the Institutional Review Board (IRB) for two terms for a total of six years. This experience was extremely valuable to my professional development, since the IRB is responsible for evaluating and approving every research protocol involving human subjects within the medical school. This experience also helped to enhance my critical thinking skills in evaluating research methodologies from a wide variety of medical disciplines. More importantly, I have acquired critical knowledge from my many patients over the past 25 years as to what treatments have been helpful. These experiences inspire me to share my thoughts and opinions on the treatment of pain.

The Scope of Pain Treatment

Because the scope of pain treatment is so extensive, I have divided this chapter into two major sections.

- Medical treatment
  - – Pharmacological approaches
  - – Invasive or surgical approaches
- Non-medical or non-invasive treatments for pain
  - – Active behavioral treatments
  - – Passive behavioral treatments

To limit the scope of this chapter, I have omitted many adjunctive and alternative therapies that are equally important in the overall treatment of pain. The most notable omission is physical and occupational therapies. The value of both PT and OT from a multidisciplinary approach is well documented and I highly recommend both.

When I discuss treatment options with patients, I use the metaphor of a toolbox. I explain that each provider will offer pain management tools for the patient's toolbox. These tools are not mutually exclusive, but additive. The more tools in your toolbox, the more effective you will be in managing your pain. Some tools may be invasive, pharmacological, or behavioral, and they are all equally important. I emphasize to the patient that any pain treatment is a partnership that requires active patient involvement. I point out that there are no "silver bullets" in terms of pain management tools. They are not necessarily curative, but if the patient is willing to work hard, they will achieve more control over their chronic pain and an improved quality of life.

Pharmacological Approaches to Pain Treatment

This section begins with a description of the World Health Organization (WHO) ladder or hierarchical scale.[38] This approach to medication management has wide acceptance in pain medicine across the United States and around the world. It proposes three successive steps, or stages, from Level I to Level III. It recommends you start with the most conservative medicines before progressing to the more potent opioid based analgesics. Level I would include your non-steroidal anti-inflammatory drugs (NSAIDS) and aspirin. Level II would include low-potency central analgesics such as codeine-based medicines. Level III is reserved for more high-potency central analgesics that are opioid based. Prescription practices vary depending on physical location, nature of practice, insurance coverage, and training levels. Plus, the efficacy or analgesia achieved is further compounded by patient variables that could include compliance issues, tolerance, and adverse reactions.

In my opinion, pharmacological approaches to pain treatment can be appropriate adjunctive tools if the prescribing physician is familiar with the patient's history of pain, type of pain, pain medicine, and contraindications related to the patient's pathology.[21]

I have worked with many prescribing pain physicians who feel that Level III opioids are not appropriate for long-term care. One pain physician I work with requires a psychosocial evaluation before prescribing long-term opioid based medicines. As a practicing pain psychologist who provides adjunctive behavioral treatment, the requirement of a psychosocial assessment appears prudent, but it is not a universally accepted approach. From a practical treatment approach, it makes sense if you know your patient's psychological profile before you enter into a long term care relationship of opioid prescribing. On the other hand, it may not be feasible in rural areas where pain psychologists are scarce. As pain psychology matures and more pain psychologists become available, I can foresee a requirement of a psychosocial evaluation becoming the rule and not the exception.

Peripheral Analgesics

The first class of pain medicines to consider are the peripheral analgesics, which are the most common and represent Level I in the analgesic ladder. Aspirin, acetaminophen, and non-steroidal anti-inflammatory drugs (NSAIDS) are the most used. All of these belong to the salicylates. NSAIDs produce pain relief by reducing the excitation of the peripheral nociceptors. According to Marchand "the reduction of prostaglandin synthesis will decrease the inflammatory response by blocking the accumulation of substances such as bradykinin and histamine which activate or sensitize the peripheral nociceptors."[21]

Therefore, NSAIDs work directly at the site of the lesion. Prostaglandins are chemical lipid mediators associated with cell membranes and are synthesized in most tissues. Unfortunately, there are well-documented adverse reactions associated with the use of NSAIDs. They may cause gastro-intestinal upset, blood issues, and neurological problems. Some patients may experience an allergic response, and these risks are higher in the older population. If the forgoing risks are an issue, then the use of acetaminophen is a safer alternative since it does not have an anti-inflammatory effect, although at higher doses it can impact the liver. A newer generation of NSAIDs have been released to the market. They are cyclooxygenase (COX). According to Marchand, there are two types, COX-1 and COX-2. COX-2 has been shown to be more effective on pain following inflammation and demonstrates less impact on the digestive system.[21]

Unfortunately, because of cardiovascular risks they have been withdrawn. The best known medicines in this group are Vioxx and Bextra. Your pain medicine provider is well aware of these implications and they will monitor reactions appropriately.

Anticonvulsants or Membrane Stabilizing Medicines

The next class of pain medicines are the anticonvulsants or the membrane stabilizing medicines. These medicines were originally developed to control seizures or epilepsy. They have since been approved for pain treatment with the most popular being Neurontin. This class of medicines is usually indicated for neuropathic pain since epilepsy and neuropathic pain are associated with changes in the sodium and calcium channels. According to Marchand, the analgesic effect of membrane stabilizers is found in their regulation of neuronal excitability in the central nervous system (CNS) by increasing inhibition or reducing excitability. They further stabilize the activity of sodium or potassium by increasing the activity of Gamma-Aminobutric Acid (GABA).

GABA is an amino acid transmitter operating in the brain, whose main function is to inhibit neuronal firing.[21] Even though this class of medicines is relatively safe, there are reported reactions associated with central effects, such as sedation, fatigue, dizziness, motor in-coordination, and vision problems.

Psychotropics or Antidepressant Medicines

The third class of medicines to be included at this level is the psychotropics or antidepressant medicines. When we discussed the role of serotonin and improving inhibition in Chapter 2, I emphasized the importance of antidepressant medicine in the pain management toolbox. Because a majority of pain patients are clinically depressed, this class of medicine has a dual purpose of improving mood and enhancing analgesic effects. My experience over the past 25 years substantiated the value of the older tricyclic medicines (TCAs), especially since shorter-acting TCAs such as desipramine and imipramine produce fewer negative side effects and do not alter sleep architecture or suppress REM sleep. An additional benefit is that they are relatively inexpensive compared to the newer antidepressants. Further, the dual acting antidepressants can be included in this class since they increase the release of serotonin and norepinephrine. Effexor and the newer version, Cymbalta, are representative of this class. There is a growing body of research supporting the use of TCAs for the following pain conditions: post-herpetic neuralgia, diabetic neuropathy, headache, rheumatoid arthritis, chronic low back pain, fibromyalgia, and cancer pain.[1]

Antidepressants are not without adverse effects. The TCAs can produce central effects such as fatigue and impaired alertness. In addition, anticholinergic effects such as dry mouth, vision problems, constipation and tremors can occur.

Opioid Therapy

In the chapter on the history of pain, I reviewed developments in the 19th century including the isolation of morphine from the opium poppy. This development led to the synthesis of many opioid-based medications that are usually divided into low-potency opiates such as codeine (Level II) and high potency opiates such as morphine (Level III).[21]

Morphine provides pain relief by inhibiting nociceptive signals within the central nervous system (CNS) and activating the descending inhibitory system. Opioid receptors are found throughout the nervous system including the periphery and within the spine.[19] Recent research indicates that the continuous infusion of morphine directly into the epidural space or cerebrospinal fluid provides direct pain relief at a lower dose.[24]

The use of opioid-based medicine has well-documented side effects at the central and peripheral locations. Well known central effects include mood changes, sedation, nausea, and respiratory depression. Peripheral adverse effects include constipation, increased pressure on the bile ducts, itching, histamine release, and urinary retention.[21] One of the most frequent issues associated with long-term use of opioid therapy is tolerance or habituation. Tolerance presents a unique problem for the prescribing pain provider, especially at higher dose levels. I recommend Scott Fishman's MD *Responsible Opioid Prescribing Guide* for a more in-depth discussion regarding this topic.[11]

Methadone has become a popular alternative to traditional opioid therapy and it deserves special mention. Methadone is a synthetic opioid that was introduced in the United States in 1947. It was originally used to treat opioid addiction. It works like the opioids but with different emphasis on the receptor subtypes. According to Chou, methadone is appropriate in the treatment of chronic non-cancer pain because of its potent analgesic effects and it is the least expensive opioid, although, methadone does have substantial risks.[7]

According to a literature review by Webster, methadone represented less than 5% of all opioids prescribed (1999–2009) but it was responsible for a third of the deaths.[37] Because of methadone's unique properties and long half-life it presents additional challenges to the provider to ensure its safe and responsible use.

Since the nature of opioid therapy presents so many potential negative outcomes, including potential addiction or dependency issues and inappropriate patient use, special considerations must be employed. The first is a provider-patient agreement or contract for long-term opioid therapy. All the pain providers with whom I have worked require some form of agreement before initiating treatment. According to Fishman, six basic elements of a patient's care should be documented in writing: (1) assessment; (2) education; (3) treatment agreement and informed consent; (4) action plans; (5) outcomes; and, (6) monitoring.[11]

As I mentioned earlier, there is a growing awareness within the pain medicine field for the re-quirement of a psychosocial evaluation before initiating long-term opioid therapy. It makes clinical sense since the provider should be fully informed of potential risks before initiating treatment rath-er than after, when it is too late.

The topic of long-term opioid therapy is beyond the scope of this chapter. I recommend an ex-cellent book on this topic published by the IASP entitled *The Pharmacology of Pain.*[1]

Surgical Approaches

Surgical treatment to help manage chronic pain can be traced back within the history of pain. The theory supporting surgical treatment is fairly straightforward. It is based on the idea that if you interrupt the nociceptive pathway by surgical section, the pain would disappear. Even though surgical techniques and approaches have improved, chronic pain has persisted and in some cases become worse. Deductive reasoning then postulated that chronic pain must be of central origin as in the example of post-amputation phantom limb pain.[12]

I discussed the complex nature of pain transmission in Chapter 2, on the nature of pain that can be traced back to the work of Henry Head. My recent clinical experience in working with patients who have gone through an ablative procedure leads me to believe that some well-selected patients will experience pain relief.

The length of pain relief can be highly variable from no relief to relief lasting months. Radical surgical procedures, such as posterior radicotomy, cordotomy, or sympathectomy, the pain signal is rarely extinguished completely. Any surgical intervention to "cure" pain is controversial at best. Spine surgery can be helpful for some, but on average only approximately 50% experience some pain relief, with moderate improvement in functional ability. About 25% of patients receive no relief at all.[4]

Failed back surgery syndrome is not well understood or accepted. It is usually a diagnosis of exclusion when a patient has experienced a poor outcome from spinal surgery. There are a number of reasons why back or spinal surgery fails. According to Oaklander and North, 2001, the most common reason is poor psychosocial status at the time of surgery.[29] This conclusion reinforces the value of a psychosocial evaluation prior to surgery. For a more complete discussion on this topic, I highly recommend the *Psychology of Spine Surgery* by Block, et al.[4]

Invasive Treatments

Next I include acupuncture and trigger point injections, since they are both invasive and are frequently used by pain providers.

Acupuncture

Acupuncture as a technique to manage pain has been around for a long time. Its origin is based in eastern medicine where it is believed that pain is the result of a disconnection between two poles of energy (yin and yang). The goal of acupuncture is to reconnect or balance the two poles of energy. Within the practice of acupuncture there exists differences of opinion regarding the placement of needles. Research findings are mixed as to the point to be stimulated.[13, 25] Reports from patients who have undergone acupuncture treatment suggests that relief is highly variable and the length of relief varies from the time needles are in place to no relief once they are removed.

Trigger Point Injections (TPIs)

Trigger Point Injections with a local anesthetic can be a useful tool if paired with physical therapy. The role of the physical therapist is to work with the patient immediately after the TPI when the trigger point is not active. The goal of the therapist is to stretch the target area while it is less painful or reactive. According to Janet Travell, trigger points vacillate between active and latent states and can persist for years.[34]

The pain relief from trigger point therapy is also highly variable and usually subsides as the anesthetic effect wears off. If the pain provider can convince the patient to use heat and stretch on a regular basis, longer lasting relief can be obtained. I also feel that deep massage or acupressure can complement the relief obtained from TPI therapy as well.

The neurophysiology of trigger points is not well understood. For a more in-depth discussion, I recommend an excellent review by Simmons.[33] Melzack found an interesting 70% correlation between the location of a trigger point and the location of an acupuncture point.[33]

Implantable Pain Technology

Before I introduce this section on implantable pain technology, I must disclose that I was a consultant to Medtronic, Inc. (Neuro Division) for 10 years. Today, I have no connection with Medtronic or any other manufacturer of medical devices. My role as a consultant was fairly unique at the time, which was based on research I published in the early 1990s while I was on the faculty at Oregon Health Sciences University. My research at the time focused on patient selection for implantable pain technology. Based on this research, I was asked to join a select faculty sponsored by Medtronic, Inc.

Spinal Cord Stimulation (SCS)

We presented numerous intensive training workshops (ITWs) around the country educating pain physicians who were interested in implantable pain technology. SCS was initially introduced by C. Norman Shealy in 1967 to help control cancer pain. Since that time there have been notable improvements in hardware and selection criteria.[4] Originally, the theory behind SCS was based on the Gate Control Theory (discussed in Chapter 2). Simply stated, SCS is based on the idea that electrical stimulation of the alpha/beta pain fibers, which in turn inhibits the alpha/delta and C fibers that, theoretically, closes the pain gate. The technique is fairly straightforward in that an electrode is placed in the epidural space by using a hollow needle. The placement of the electrode is based on the patient's pain presentation. Prior to this trial the patient will undergo psychosocial evaluation to rule out risk factors that may interfere with a successful outcome.[4] If the patient is an appropriate candidate, the next step is a trial period where the patient goes home and tries out the SCS. The trial period can vary depending on the implanting physician, but it usually lasts from 5–7 days. At the end of the trial period, the patient will meet with the implanting physician to determine if the trial was a success. The criteria for success will vary with each implanting physician.

Sometimes the results of the trial are mixed. The patient may experience relief in certain places, but it may not cover all of the painful areas. In this case, the patient and the implanting physician have to consider the benefits of partial pain relief before proceeding to final implantation. As I mentioned earlier, outcome research is mixed with published reports indicating 50–75% relief for those patients proceeding to permanent implantation. For an excellent review, I recommend a number of articles. Please refer to references 28, 30, and 5.

Direct Infusion

The other major form of implantable pain technology is direct infusion or neuraxial drug administration. This form of therapy was initially approved for cancer pain, but has now been approved for benign or non-cancer pain. It allows opioid based medicines to be administered directly to opioid receptors by passing the blood brain barrier. This form of administration allows for a smaller amount of medicine to achieve similar or improved results without the side effects of oral administration.[9]

Non-medical/Non-invasive Treatments

Transcutaneous Electrical Nerve Stimulation (TENS)

Transcutaneous Electrical Nerve Stimulation is a widely-used non-invasive treatment. TENS is theoretically based on the Gate Control model of pain since it inhibits the pain signal through the stimulation of non-nociceptive pain fibers. In practical clinical terms, the theory is based on the assumption that electrical peripheral stimulation of a specific region produces a localized analgesic effect. Keep in mind that this is also the basis for muscle stimulation techniques so I will not include additional discussion of this procedure. TENS approaches can be grouped into two categories:

- Conventional TENS which is based on stimulating non-painful nerve fibers
- Acupuncture-like TENS that works on stimulating painful nerve fibers

Conventional TENS uses high frequency, low intensity stimulation to produce paresthesia; spontaneous or provoked abnormal sensation (non-painful) without producing pain. Research supporting the clinical use of TENS is mixed.[10, 22, 27] My clinical experience with patients suggests that for some patients it can be a useful tool and therefore it is worth a trial.

One caveat pointed out by Marchand is that caffeine appears to block the optimal effect of TENS even at low doses. Therefore, it is important to limit coffee, caffeine-based teas, chocolate, and colas.[22, 23] In addition, there is evidence suggesting that opioid-based medicine may produce a cross-tolerance in acupuncture-like TENS, but not to conventional TENS.[17]

Behavioral Treatments

In this section, I introduce behavioral techniques, passive and active, that have empirical support. In my own clinical practice, I will include the use of relaxation therapy if it is appropriate. I have found that not all pain patients will respond to relaxation therapy, so it takes some flexibility on the part of the provider to determine if relaxation therapy is appropriate. If the patient agrees to actively pursue relaxation therapy, I will augment this training with the use of biofeedback. I introduced biofeedback in Chapter 3, so it is not necessary to repeat that information. I consider the use of relaxation therapy and biofeedback to be an active form of therapy, but I will also include passive techniques as described below.

Deep Breathing Technique

I will describe the treatment algorithm that I follow in my own practice. If sympathetic reactivity appears to be contributory to the patient's pain experience, I initially instruct the patient in the technique of deep breathing or breathing from the diaphragm. It is best if the patient is wearing loose-fitting clothing and if they are wearing a belt to undo it. I start by asking the patient to take a deep breath through the nose, expanding their chest, holding their breath for a few seconds, then exhaling through the mouth and emptying their lungs. I have them practice a couple of breaths with their eyes closed and repeating a mantra to themselves as they exhale.

I let them pick their own mantra. The one I use is "relax." I explain that when they are under stress or experiencing a pain episode, most patients will revert to shallow breathing or holding their breath completely. At this point. I may add visualization or imagining their pain as Swiss cheese and to breathe through the pain as you would breathe through the holes in the Swiss cheese. To enhance the emptying of the lungs on exhale, I suggest another visualization of blowing up a balloon, blowing their pain, stress, and worries into the balloon. I then instruct them to let the balloon float up into the sky until it disappears since there is no string attached to the balloon. It is important to caution the patient to be well supported when they practice this technique, since they will sometimes feel lightheaded due to the change of CO_2 in their blood stream.

Progressive Relaxation

Once the patient has mastered the deep breathing technique, I introduce progressive relaxation. I should mention that not every patient is appropriate for progressive relaxation since it is a technique based on isometric contraction of a muscle group. I will also caution the patient not to contract muscle groups if it produces pain, since we do not want to trigger a muscle spasm. I instruct them to avoid these groups and we will cover them at a later date when we progress to visualization techniques.

Progressive relaxation was introduced in the 1920s by Edmund Jacobson and it is sometimes referred to as the Jacobson Technique.[14] Jacobson's premise was that if he could relax your muscles, your brain would then relax. As you relax your muscles, sympathetic arousal will also relax, thereby lowering your pain levels. Early in my career, I would personally talk the patient through the various muscle groups. Today, I use professionally made CDs that are conveniently available. My favorite CDs are produced by Miller and Halpern and I will include specific recommendations in the reference section of this chapter.[26]

I enhance the relaxation response by adding deep breathing to coincide with the tensing of the muscle groups. I accomplish this by instructing the patient to take a deep breath as they tense the muscle and then exhale as they relax the muscle, letting the tension float away.

Augmented Techniques

As I mentioned earlier, I will augment the relaxation experience with the use of a temperature thermistor, which they can take with them and practice in their own environment. I described this approach in Chapter 3, so I will not go into depth other than to mention that most patients can increase their skin temperature a couple of degrees after 20–30 minutes with the above approach. The use of temperature feedback reinforces the mind-body connection and provides a simple method of demonstrating sympathetic reactivity. Progressive relaxation is a fairly straightforward technique that I have used on a wide age range of patients from children to older adults.

Before I progress to the next stage of relaxation training, I assess the patient's openness to more abstract techniques. I have found Auke Tellegen's Absorption Scale to be helpful in selecting patients for more suggestive therapies including autogenics and self-hypnosis.[35] Additionally, I will ask the patient two questions that are from the Harvard Hypnotic Scales.[32] First, can you dictate your dream activity, and second, can you set your internal clock to awaken you at a certain time without the use of an external clock?

If the patient can answer yes to at least one, or both, of these questions my experience tells me they are probably good candidates for suggestive relaxation techniques. In addition, I highly recommend the book by Herbert Benson, MD, *The Relaxation Response*, to complement the patient's knowledge base. It is very readable and explains in basic terms the importance of controlling your physiological arousal by mastering the relaxation response.[3]

If the patient does well with progressive relaxation and they are open and motivated to learn a more abstract and powerful technique, I introduce Autogenic Therapy. Autogenics was introduced by Luthe and is based on self-phrasing and visualization.[20] Based on my clinical experience, I have found it difficult for the patient to initiate Autogenics without some experience with relaxation or meditation training. In practical terms, Autogenics is more effective if the patient can quiet their sympathetic arousal before initiating the self-phrasing technique. I share with the patient that as we relax, our brain becomes more open or absorbent to our own suggestions. It enhances concentration and narrows focus.

I consider Autogenic therapy a form of initial self-hypnosis. If the patient is progressing at this point in therapy, I encourage the use of positive self-affirmations which is a form of self-hypnotic suggestion. In other words, when you give yourself a positive self-affirmation in a deeply relaxed state, it increases the probability that it will become a self-fulfilling prophecy. The next step in my clinical algorithm is the addition of a self-hypnotic induction procedure to achieve a deeper state of relaxation. The induction procedure I use the most is the image of an elevator (the old fashioned type, not the high-speed ones we have now, which would be counterproductive). When in a relaxed state, I ask the patient to imagine standing in front of an elevator door, usually on the tenth floor. The door opens, they get on alone, the door closes and they push the down button. They focus on the floor indicator hand that, like a clock, moves down as the elevator descends slowly floor by floor. As each floor passes they take a deep breath and as they exhale, repeat to themselves a mantra or the word "relax." When they reach the ground floor, the door opens and they walk out in a deeply-relaxed state.

A variation on the induction procedure that I have found helpful in promoting deeper and more restful sleep is to imagine your bed waiting for you when the door opens and as you crawl into bed, repeat the following affirmation, "I will have a deep and restful sleep" and to repeat this affirmation as you drop off to sleep. If the patient awakes during the night, they can repeat the procedure to help fall asleep faster and achieve deeper sleep. Personally, I do not recommend traditional hypnosis since my treatment philosophy is based on giving the patient skills or tools that they can take with them without fostering a dependence on me to guide them. If the reader is interested in hypnosis as a treatment tool, I recommend Mark Jensen's book, *Hypnosis for Chronic Pain Management*.[15]

Cognitive Behavioral Therapy (CBT)

Before I introduce Cognitive Behavioral Therapy (CBT) for pain, a brief personal history may be helpful for the reader to appreciate the perspective and evaluation of how behavioral therapy became the therapy of choice for chronic pain. When I was in graduate school in the 70s, behavior therapy was becoming more accepted.

It was based on the early work of B. F. Skinner that was introduced in Chapters 2 and 3. Early behavior therapy is founded in operant learning theory that assumes our behavior is shaped by the consequences we experience in our environment. When Fordyce introduced the term "pain behavior" it was a logical extension of operant learning theory. I still use operant learning techniques in my practice. According to Keefe and Lefebvre, operant learning processes are likely to play an important role in shaping and maintaining pain behaviors that are maladaptive.[16]

The ABCs or circular model of pain behavior that I introduced in Chapter 3 is based on operant learning principles. First there is the Antecedent or trigger (A) that leads to the pain Behavior (B) and then the Consequent results (C).

My doctoral dissertation examined the role of self-monitoring; does charting a behavior modify or influence a behavior? The results of my research indicated that the act of keeping track of behavior is a reinforcing event that will modify behavior. Using this finding, I encourage pain patients to monitor their ABCs on a daily basis and if the patient is willing to take this data a step further, to chart this information in the form of a graph.

I request that the patient post this information, usually on the refrigerator where the entire family or support system can observe. This act of public disclosure adds additional power or therapeutic effect to the entire self-monitoring exercise. I also ask the patient to bring their data or graph to each session so that we can troubleshoot and discuss treatment options.

In the 1970s, Beck introduced the idea that a person's thoughts or cognitions can exert a significant impact on their mood, behavior, and physiology.[2] This idea was a logical next step in the evolution of behavior therapy that led to what we now call Cognitive Behavioral Therapy (CBT). CBT techniques help patients modify or change negative thought patterns that contribute to pain behavior and eventual depression.[18, 36]

CBT techniques are also designed to promote positive coping strategies as they relate to pain. Specific techniques can include cognitive restructuring or reframing, problem solving, distraction and relapse prevention. There is a growing body of empirical research supporting CBT as applied to a variety of pain conditions that has established CBT as the behavioral therapy of choice.[8]

Summary

It is a difficult task to cover all treatments for chronic pain, therefore, I have focused on treatments that are supported by empirical research. The intent of this chapter was to cover a variety of treatment options that are complementary from a multidisciplinary approach. I have included some of my personal approaches and techniques that have evolved out of many years as a pain provider.

I have also omitted newer alternative treatments that sound promising, but are not yet well supported by empirical data. The March 7, 2011 issue of *TIME* magazine devoted considerable space to chronic pain, including their cover page entitled, "Understanding Pain."

If the reader is interested in newer alternative treatments such as the healing power of touch and mirror therapy for phantom limb pain, it is worth your time to read the article presented. That issue of TIME magazine is available online.[31]

Finally, if the reader is interested in more specific techniques mentioned in this chapter, I would highly recommend the workbook by Margaret Caudill, MD, PhD, *Managing Pain Before it Manages You* (3rd Edition).[6]

The foregoing four chapters represent the core chapters, or the first major section of this book. The next section will focus on specific areas of pain with the concluding section devoted to case studies.

Chapter

5 Pain and Sleep

*He had no curiosity, sensation and emotion had left him. He was no longer
susceptible to pain. Stomach and nerves had gone to sleep.*
–JACK LONDON, *Love of Life* (1907)

The Relationship Between Pain and Sleep

Introduction

IN 2011, I AUTHORED AN ARTICLE in *Practical Pain Management* entitled "Pain and Sleep: A
Delicate Balance."[28] The main premise of the article is that a strong relationship exists between pain
and sleep and that it is reciprocal. I also pointed out that a delicate balance exists between pain and
sleep and that impacts the patient's overall homeostatic balance.

In this chapter, I will present a more in depth look at the interrelationship of pain and sleep by
presenting a review of the growing body of research that reflects an increasing awareness of this
interrelationship. Further, we will explore the causality of the pain and sleep association, including
the mechanisms that may help explain this association. We will discuss treatment options that are
relevant to both sleep and pain.

In earlier chapters I mentioned that pain is a signal of bodily harm and that sleep is a behavior-
ally regulated drive that helps maintain homeostasis. If homeostasis is compromised by pain that
results in sleep disruption, negative consequences will impact health and well-being.

A recent critical review on the association of sleep and pain pointed out the growing research
evidence that supports the sleep-pain association.[11]

This article proposed two fundamental questions. First, are pain and sleep reciprocally or unidirectionally related? Second, what mechanisms account for this association between sleep and pain?
Prior to the Finan article published in 2013, Smith and Haythornthwaite published an excellent
review on sleep and pain in 2004. Their review suggested that pain and sleep were in a reciprocal
relationship.[34] Since their 2004 review, there are more prospective studies, with more longitudinal
data, more pain conditions and larger epidemiological studies that have all contributed to further
understanding of the pain and sleep association.

The major focus of this chapter will be what Finan, et al, identified in their 2013 article. They selected
17 well-designed studies that were conducted between 2005 and 2012 that attempt to answer the
two questions: Are pain and sleep reciprocal or unidirectional and what are the mechanisms? With
respect to the first question, they included studies that focused on the unidirectional effect of sleep
on future pain. They included three large longitudinal studies that indicted that elevated insomnia

symptoms increase the risk of headache with a long-term follow-up ranging from 1 to 12 years.[3, 22, 27]

It is important to point out that the research was selective to tension type headache and not migraine. An additional large population study of Norwegian women (N=15,350) with an eleven year follow up found that sleep disorders predicted fibromyalgia 10 years later.[25] The authors of this study estimated that 2/3 of the sample that were diagnosed with fibromyalgia was explained by preexisting sleep problems.

The 2013 review by Finan concluded that other prospective studies that suggested that sleep problems increase the risk of chronic pain in pain free individuals, worsens the long-term prognosis of existing headache and chronic musculoskeletal pain and influences daily fluctuations in clinical pain. Conversely, they also mention that good sleep appears to improve the long-term prognosis of individuals with chronic pain conditions.[11]

Next, Finan, et al, evaluated recent prospective studies assessing bidirectional effects of sleep and pain. They proposed that a trend has emerged suggesting that sleep disturbances may predict pain to a greater degree than pain predicts sleep problems. Their broad analysis of data suggests that sleep and pain appear to be a reciprocally related, but a closer analysis suggests that poor sleep may have a stronger influence on the experience of chronic pain.[11]

The current growing body of research strongly suggests, at the clinical level, that sleep quality should be included in the initial assessment of all patients who present with chronic pain. In my opinion, this is not a difficult task. For the past 25 years I have included interview questions that assess the quality of the patient's sleep. (See Chapter 3 on the assessment of pain.) If I determine that a sleep problem exists, I will ask the patient to fill out a sleep log that covers one week. Further, I will include the Epworth Sleepiness Scale (available free of charge online).[17] The ESS scale is easy to administer. It takes ten minutes to administer and it provides additional information to help rule out if a sleep disorder exists. I will include this information in my report back to the referring physician so they can decide if a formal sleep study is indicated.

Now that I have shown that pain and sleep go together, either reciprocally or bidirectionally, we will examine the scope or prevalence. The numbers for chronic pain were presented in Chapter 2. Based on large community studies from around the world, one finding consistently stands out: chronic pain appears to be the main reason why patients do not sleep well. These effects includes the criteria for insomnia (defined as difficulty initiating sleep, disrupted sleep, early morning awakenings, and unrefreshing sleep. Because there is no uniform methodology in the pain/sleep epidemiological studies, the estimated prevalence is quite variable ranging from 23% in Europe to a high of 89% in the US.

Below is a summary of research findings on sleep disturbances in chronic pain conditions:
1. The prevalence of sleep problems in patients who suffer from chronic pain is higher than the general population. It appears more common in arthritic conditions.

2. The percentage of pain patients who describe sleep problems varies from 50% to 89%.

3. The most common reported sleep problem in pain patients is insomnia.

4. The most common sleep findings in chronic pain patients include sleep fragmentations,

decreased sleep efficiency, and reduced slow-wave sleep.

5. Alpha-delta intrusions during non-REM sleep are not specific to fibromyalgia. They are also found in other types of pain conditions and non-pain subjects.

6. A number of pain patients also report other sleep disorders such as apnea and restless leg syndrome.[6]

It is important to keep in mind that the research supports the fact that pain and sleep are interrelated, but that the relationship is complex due to the many factors that can influence both processes.

Now that the foundation has been presented that sleep and pain are reciprocally related, both bidirectionally and unidirectionally, the next step should be a discussion concerning the nature of sleep. The nature of pain is covered in Chapter 2. The following section will cover the types and patterns of sleep, how sleep is generated by the brain and the role that sleep plays in the individual's overall functioning. It is important to understand the mechanics and physiology of sleep to be able to appreciate the interrelationship of pain and sleep on the physical and behavioral levels.

The Nature of Sleep

What is sleep and why is it so important to the pain patient and the treatment of the pain experience? The average individual spends a considerable amount of time sleeping. About one third of our life is spent in this endeavor. In the past, it was thought that sleep was quiet time for the brain and body to recuperate from the demands of the day. Recent sleep research has refined that notion and has discovered that sleep is a carefully controlled and highly regulated series of states that occur in a cyclical fashion each night. Sleep is critical in maintaining homeostasis, which reinforces that fact that we need uninterrupted sleep to survive and cope with the demands of every day life. The need for quality sleep is critically important for the pain patient who deals with the additional demands that pain imposes on maintaining homeostatic balance.

Sleep is divided into two separate and distinct states: non-rapid eye movement (non-REM) and rapid eye movement (REM) sleep. Both are equally important in maintaining physical and mental homeostasis. When a patient undergoes a sleep study, brain wave activity is monitored by an electroencephalogram (EEG). This information helps the sleep physician determine the quality and quantity of both non-REM and REM sleep.

Non-REM sleep is divided into four stages: Stage I and II are considered "light sleep" and Stages III and IV are considered "deep sleep". As we progress from Stage I to Stage IV, brain wave activity slows down, as measured by the EEG from active beta wave to slow delta wave sleep. Non-REM sleep is important for both brain and body restoration. REM sleep is considered active sleep because brain activity and EEG patterns are similar to brain activity when we are awake. During REM our muscle systems are inactive unlike heart rate, breathing and blood pressure, which are highly variable. Also during REM sleep we experience story life dream activity. In my opinion, it is our ability to dream that is critical in maintaining mental homeostasis. Dreaming allows us to problem solve the demands of life and when REM sleep is disrupted mental disturbances can result. I will revisit this issue later on in this chapter when pain and sleep medicines are reviewed.

As I mentioned earlier, sleep stages are cyclical. REM and non-REM sleep alternate throughout our time asleep. Below is a summary of our sleep cycles and stages:

Stage I sleep (non-REM) lasts about 1-10 minutes before Stage II begins.

Stage III is slower wave activity and lasts for only a few minutes before Stage IV appears.

When more than 50% of brain activity (EEG patterns) is slow wave activity, it is classified as Stage IV non-REM sleep.

After about 20–40 minutes of Stage IV sleep we progress into lighter sleep, moving into Stage III, then Stage II and finally REM sleep, which lasts for about 5 minutes.

This cycle continues to alternate throughout the night finally ending in REM sleep. According to Carskadon and Dement, the first half of the night is usually non-REM sleep (Stages III and IV) with brief REM sleep periods. As sleep progresses, Stages III and IV decrease and Stage II becomes more evident (non-REM). REM sleep becomes longer reaching the maximum during the last third of the night. REM sleep periods can range from 4 – 6 minutes depending upon the length of sleep. Sleep cycles change throughout the total sleep time with an approximate length of 90 minutes. Healthy adults spend about 75% to 80% of sleep time in non-REM sleep and about 20% to 25% in REM sleep. It is important to appreciate how fragile and critical this cyclic progression is upon our ability to cope with life's demands and maintain our mental and physical balance.

My own experience in working with a sleep center as a behavioral consultant allowed me to examine

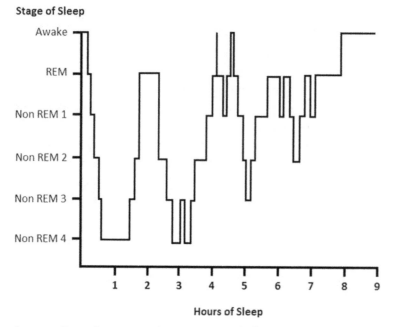

sleep studies of patients who experienced chronic pain. I observed consistent patterns of excessive Stage I and Stage II sleep with little or no Stage III or Stage IV slow wave sleep. This observation made sense to me since pain patients will experience painful episodes throughout the night when they roll over or spend too much time in one position. This observation is probably more relevant to myofascial and joint pain as compared to some neuropathic pain conditions. Neuropathic pain can occur independent of movement and is usually described as a burning sensation.

If the sleep cycle is interrupted by pain, the patient will recycle to Stage I or II and do not progress on to deeper, slow wave sleep. This pattern will repeat itself throughout the night, which results in a continuous sleep debt that produces a constant state of daytime fatigue. As days of fatigue accumulate, additional stress is experienced and the patient's pain threshold will be negatively compromised. In addition, if the pain patient does not sleep well they will usually spend more time in bed usually in light or non-restorative sleep. This pattern is also found in depressed patients with or without pain.

Next, we need to consider the neurological control of sleep and the interesting overlap that exists with the neural control of pain and sleep. Recent research findings suggest that specific brain regions play a critical role in sleep regulation. This is also true for the regulation of pain.[29] Work conducted by Saper found that damage to the anterior hypothalamus caused severe insomnia.[32] His findings suggest that the hypothalamus is involved in controlling both waking and sleeping states, which is also true for the control of pain. Further, Saper's work pointed out that the hypothalamus and the basal forebrain generate non-REM sleep. It is relevant to point out that both of these areas contain active GABAergic neurons, which have an important role in the control of pain and sleep. These GABAergic neurons are sensitive to change in body temperature that forms a "sleep switch" that turns sleep on and off.[32] These findings suggest that GABA is interrelated to both sleep and pain at the neurophysiological level.

REM sleep is controlled primarily by the brain stem which also overlaps the neural control of pain. Additional recent research has indicated that dopamine may be involved in sleep regulation. As I mentioned in Chapter 2, dopamine is also involved in the regulation of pain and mood. Dysregulation of the dopamine system may lead to persistent insomnia or sleepiness.[23, 37]

The above research findings suggest that pain and sleep are interrelated with dopamine levels. This association has important implications for the pharmacological treatment of the patient who experiences both pain and disrupted sleep.

Treatment Options

In this next section we will review the treatment options available for both sleep and pain. First, I will review pharmaceutical options that have implications for both pain and sleep. Second, I will review behavioral approaches that are empirically based and appropriate for both pain and sleep. I recommend to the reader that they review Chapter 4 for background information on the treatment of pain.

The most frequently prescribed pain medicines are opiod based, both short acting and long term continuous acting. A growing body of research has repeatedly demonstrated that opioids disrupt sleep architecture and inhibit REM sleep.[21, 1] As I mentioned earlier the balance between REM and non-REM sleep is critical in maintaining homeostasis. REM sleep is especially critical in maintaining optimal mental health. Consistent research findings have suggested that sleep disruption is an unwanted opioid side effect that results in a lower pain threshold.[1, 30]

Unfortunately, there are few studies examining the effects of NSAIDs on sleep in either healthy subjects or chronic pain patients. There are a few studies that have examined this issue that suggest that NSAIDs and acetaminophen do not appear to affect sleep architecture in healthy human subjects.[2] A small study of patients with rheumatoid arthritis that were prescribed Tenoxicam (NSAID) for 90 days reported a 50% reduction in joint pain with no altered sleep architecture.[20]

The results of antidepressant research on pain and sleep are mixed. The older tricyclic (TCAs) based medicines suggest that some of the TCAs suppress REM sleep, especially amitriptyline.[36] The newer serotonin reuptake inhibitors (SSRIs) have also been found to inhibit REM sleep.[36] When comparing the old TCAs and the newer SSRIs on sleep alone, the newer SSRIs appear to have little effect on sleep architecture excluding REM sleep, but it is unknown if they have a favorable effect on pain. Conversely, there is research supporting the use of TCAs in the treatment of neuropathic and muscle pain.[31] The one antidepressant that appears to have little or no effect on SWS or REM sleep time is nefazadone.[33]

Based on my clinical experience as a pain psychologist, I have found that a trial of the shorter acting TCAs at a small or homeopathic dose level at bedtime to be helpful. By starting with a small dose (10–20 mg) of the shorter acting TCAs you minimize unwanted side effects and if initially helpful, you can titrate upwards slowly. Further, I have found over the years that prescribing physicians often start with too big of a dose of TCAs which produce immediate unwanted side effects that result in the patient discontinuing the trial prematurely without fully knowing if the TCA would have been helpful.

In Chapter 2, I reviewed the importance of antidepressants in contributing to the descending inhibition of the pain signal. I have previously pointed out that the majority of pain patients are clinically depressed. Therefore, based on these two findings a trial of an appropriate antidepressant medicine appears warranted for the pain patient who also experiences a sleep disorder.

Recent research has supported the use of antiepileptic medicines in the treatment of neuropathic pain and other chronic pain disorders.[7] It appears that some of the older antiepileptic medicines appear to have negative side effects on sleep architecture, but the newer medicines appear to have minimal or even beneficial effects on sleep quality.[4] Both gabapentin and pregabalin have been found to increase SWS without affecting REM sleep.[15]

There is a growing body of sleep research emphasizing the important role of circadian rhythms and the maintenance of homeostatic balance. As I mentioned earlier homeostatic balance is especially important for the pain patient who does not sleep well. Therefore, we need to briefly discuss the role that the circadian clock plays in influencing the quality of sleep time. If you disrupt the circadian rhythms in humans it will have a negative impact on maintaining homeostatic balance that includes the pain experience. Again it is interesting to note the neural overlap between pain and the regulation of circadian rhythms and sleep by the anterior hypothalamus. More specifically the suprachiasmatic nucleus (SCN) which is beyond the scope of this chapter, but I will provide an excellent review of this topic for readers who are interested in this topic.[9] The pineal gland, which produces melatonin, is regulated by the SCN, with the exposure to light/dark cycle being the main synchronizer. Melatonin is stimulated by darkness and inhibited by light. According to Doghramji this process is controlled by two melatonin receptors located in the SCN.

One of the primary determinants that influence the quality of our sleep is homeostatically regulated.[32] This physiological drive for sleep progresses during the day (light) and then dissipated during sleep (dark). Further, it is believed that this homeostatic drive for sleep is genetically influenced.[12] During the evening melatonin increases which allows sleep to occur. The other neuromodulator that affects homeostatic sleep drive is adenosine which is accumulated during the day and eventually activates sleep-promoting neurons.[9]

Melatonin is the primary neurohormone of the pineal gland and plays a critical role in regulating circadian rhythms. Light transmission from the retina stimulates neural signals into the anterior hypothalamus and the SCN. These signals are then relayed to the pineal gland. Brzezinski found in humans that the nocturnal rise in melatonin begins after the onset of darkness, peaks in the middle of the sleep period (between 2 and 4 am) and then gradually falls during the second half of the night.[4] In addition, melatonin has been found to induce sedation and lower core body temperature.[19]

Even though the research is mixed on the effectiveness of melatonin, I have found in my own practice that for some patients it has been helpful in promoting sleep. It is relatively inexpensive and it is classified by the FDA as a dietary supplement and no serious side effects have been associated with the use of melatonin. It should be noted that melatonin has a short half-life, therefore, I recommend to my patients that they try a sustained release formulation. They should take it approximately 30 minutes before bedtime with dose ranges from 1 mg to 10 mg. Also keep in mind that as we age our natural melatonin levels decrease so that age becomes an additional factor to consider. This decrease in melatonin levels especially in the senior population is felt by some sleep researchers to conclude that this may be one factor why as we age our sleep quality decreases.

In 2005 the FDA approved a prescription form of melatonin (Ramelton) for the treatment of insomnia, especially for difficulty with sleep onset. Initial research results suggest that it does work faster as compared to melatonin and that it exhibits a longer half-life.[18] In one well controlled study with varying dose levels of 4, 8, 16 and 32 mg all dose levels showed significant results in lowering sleep onset time.[10] Because it is a relatively new prescribed sleep aid, it is incumbent upon the prescribing physician to be well informed, as there are reported serious side effects. The limited scope of this chapter does not permit me to include all of the pharmo-therapies for insomnia. I recommend to the reader an excellent article contained in the supplement to the *Journal of Clinical Sleep Medicine* by David N. Neubauer.[26]

To conclude this section on the analgesic use and subsequent effect on sleep architecture I will present the following summary table from Cairns.[4]

Drug Class	Light Sleep	SWS	REM sleep
Opioids	Increase	Decrease	Decrease
NSAIDs	No Effect	Decrease	No Effect
TCAs	Drug Specific	Increase	No Effect
Antiepileptics	No Effect	Drug Specific	Drug Specific
Cannabinoids	Increase	Drug Specific	Drug Specific
NMDA Antagonists	Increase	Increase	Decrease

Behavioral Treatment for Pain and Sleep

There is a growing body of research supporting the association between pain and sleep that includes a number of cognitive-behavioral factors. These identified factors are mood disturbance, inactivity, conditioned hyper-arousal and presleep cognitive rumination.[14, 24, 34, 35]

Cognitive-behavioral therapies for pain and insomnia usually include relaxation training augmented by biofeedback, coping skills training, cognitive therapy, increasing activity levels and goal setting. There are newer promising cognitive based therapies that include mindfulness meditation, movement therapy and action commitment therapy (ACT). There is an ongoing debate within the pain psychology community regarding these "newer" therapies. Are they a new generation of cognitive behavioral therapy (CBT) or do they represent additional tools under the umbrella of cognitive behavioral therapy? In may opinion they represent the latter. They appear to me to be additional tools that the pain patient can add to their pain management tool box. Because they have not met the "test of time" they will not be included in this section. For a more detailed discussion of the above issues, I recommend an excellent review and discussion by Jensen and Turk in the *American Psychologist,* special issue, on chronic pain and psychology.[16]

When a patient in my practice is identified as having both pain and sleep issues, I also use a behavioral technique that includes a thorough discussion of sleep hygiene and the use of a sleep log. Sleep hygiene consists of basic information to improve sleep quality and the use of a sleep log was mentioned in Chapter 3 on assessment and Chapter 4 on treatment. As I mentioned previously, self-monitoring of any behavior is reactive or therapeutic, and in this example, keeping track of sleep behavior becomes part of the therapy. An additional tool that has become available is a portable actigraph, which can be worn on the wrist and is fairly inexpensive. The information gained from using an actigraph can provide useful assessment information and also become part of the treatment in the form of self-monitoring.

I would like to reinforce a consistent clinical feature that is common to both pain and insomnia. Psychophysiological arousal is a key component that is common in both conditions. Psychophysiological arousal for me is the same as sympathetic reactivity and/or clinical anxiety. When a patient is described as anxious I usually assess sympathetic reactivity by the use of a skin temperature thermistor, which will usually reflect cooler skin readings suggesting vasoconstriction.

If the patient is cold in the extremities at bedtime, it will take longer for the patient to fall asleep. I have also found in my own practice that if the patient is cold in the extremities, they will usually report higher pain levels. Keep in mind skin temperature or blood flow is relative. Individually, we have a physiological window that will vary depending on our level of sympathetic reactivity. I have found that skin temperatures below 80 degrees are clinically significant. Mid 80s suggest moderate sympathetic reactivity and low 90s are ideal. If I can raise a patient's skin temperature by a couple of degrees using relaxation therapy augmented by temperature biofeedback they will usually report lower pain levels.

This finding is also true for sleep. I instruct the patient to use relaxation techniques while in bed, check their skin thermistor for increased skin temperature. I also instruct the patient to use positive affirmations of a deep and restful sleep as they progress to a deeper state of relaxation. If they awake during the night I encourage them to repeat the above sequence. More importantly, if they can achieve more restful sleep with behavioral techniques without the use of a sleep aid (medication) they will feel an enhanced sense of self-control or self-efficacy. Keep in mind we are not trying to duplicate core temperature, just skin temperature, which is reflective of sympathetic reactivity.

Further, I propose that control of sympathetic reactivity should be the "gold standard" for all CBT therapies whether it be progressive relaxation, autogenics, self-hypnosis or mindfulness meditation. Also for the provider, keep in mind that one technique or approach may not fit all of your patients, so it is important to remain flexible and patient as you explore various treatment options.

Next, I would like to include a discussion on the relationship of pain and dream activity. Historically there are a few published anecdotal reports from the late 19th century and early 20th century. These early reports focused on the sensory experiences that could occur in dreams. According to Zadia and Manzini, reference to physical pain was absent from everyday dream reports or were indirectly incorporated into the dream when generated by an external stimulus.[38]

Today we know that dream activity usually occurs during REM sleep, but it can also occur during other sleep stages. Research findings from sleep studies suggest that sensory stimuli applied during REM can influence dream activity. Further, these sleep studies suggest that patients who participated (over 300 dream reports) do not incorporate physical pain in their dreams. The authors conclude that based on these reports the dreaming mind is unable to incorporate physical pain sensations.[38]

Recent work by Antonio Damasio explored the relationship of dreaming and consciousness. Damasio found that consciousness is also depressed during REM sleep. But during REM sleep dream content can enter consciousness by learning or subsequent recall.[8] In my opinion, REM sleep and dreaming are important for the pain patient in maintaining a sense of self and promoting mental homeostasis. The act of dreaming protects us from painful experiences so it is not surprising that the pain patient would not include pain into their dream content.

I have found in my own clinical practice that some patients can dictate their dream activity. This can be a useful tool in helping the patient cope with their pain. I will often ask the patient what are the themes of their dream activity and can they construct positive approaches to cope with their pain on a daily basis. The use of relaxation therapy can be helpful in the patient's home environment.

I will ask the patient to dream about some of the goals we are focusing on in therapy and how they can improve the quality of their life.

In Chapter 3, I discussed the work of Auke Tellegen and the "absorbent mind." In a deep relaxed state, the mind is more open or absorbent to self-directed thoughts.

Summary

Hopefully, this chapter reinforced the importance that quality sleep is critical for the pain patient in maintaining mental and physical homeostasis. There is a growing awareness within the pain community that sound restorative sleep is important for the pain patient to cope with persistent discomfort on a daily basis. We now have recent evidence that indicates that pain and sleep are a reciprocal interdependent relationship. Further, recent research has indicated that poor sleep can predict pain in certain conditions and that poor sleep compounds the pain experience. Therefore, it is clinically important for all pain providers to include an assessment of sleep quality for all patients living with chronic pain.

Early in my career, I was fortunate to attend a week-long sleep workshop conducted by Peter Hauri, PhD. Dr. Hauri is no longer with us, but during his long career as a sleep psychologist, he was considered a preeminent authority on sleep disorders. For those of you who are interested in a comprehensive sleep program, I highly recommend his book, *No More Sleepless Nights*.[13] There is also a workbook available that complements his approach to improving the quality of sleep.

Chapter

6 Age and Pain

Age is an issue of mind over matter. If you don't mind, it doesn't matter.
–Mark Twain

The central topic of this chapter is age and how age influences the perception of the pain experience. We will focus on the extremes of the age continuum from children to the older adult. We will examine the role of age as it relates to social and physiological development, cognitive processing and coping skills. This chapter will also include a discussion of the role of the caregiver for both children and the older adult.

Pain in Children

In 2012, the American Pain Society Task Force on Pediatric Chronic Pain defined chronic pain as recurrent or persistent pain lasting longer than normal tissue healing time, approximately three to six months.[2]

Not long ago, it was believed that children did not feel pain. This belief was based on research from the 20th century that argued in order for pain to be perceived, the myelination of the nerve pathways must be complete.[41] In 1941, research by McGraw stated that because of the incomplete development of the cerebral cortex, children were incapable of any memory before the age of six months.[30] Based on these findings, it was believed that children rarely needed analgesic medicine after surgery including the use of opioids.

Today we know that nociceptors are in place from the 20th week of intrauterine life and that the peripheral pathways, although not yet myelinated, are in place before the end of the embryonic period.[3, 5] Therefore, we now know that all of the neuro-physiological structures involved in processing the pain signal are in place several weeks before birth. Further, based on recent research, it is now believed that the newborn is more vulnerable to pain as compared to the adult.[4, 29, 35]

Children can experience a wide variety of painful conditions including cancer, arthritis, diabetic neuropathies, complex regional pain syndromes, fibromyalgia, irritable bowel syndrome, and headache, to name a few. For those of you who are interested in a more complete discussion on the types of pain in childhood, I would recommend an excellent chapter by Schechter, et al.[39]

Because of the inconsistent criteria used in assessing pain in children, prevalence numbers vary widely. According to Perquim, during childhood the most frequent pain conditions are abdominal, musculoskeletal and headache pain.[34] The best estimate of moderate to severe pain in childhood is 5%.[20]

The central question that needs to be explored is how children experience pain. Recent thinking has identified three components involved in childhood pain: the directive, discriminative, and cognitive components.[5] According to Marchand, the directive component is transmitted by the C fibers, which represent slow and diffuse pain. The discriminative component is transmitted by the A-delta fibers, which are the faster, smaller myelinated fibers. The cognitive component refers to the brain and its capacity to understand the pain experience. The cognitive component is influenced by family, culture, education, and previous painful experiences.[26]

In order to better understand how these components interface, we need to briefly review the major stages of child development. According to Piaget, the major stages of development are completed by age fourteen. The following outline indicates the major points for each stage of development.

Stages of Development

The Sensorimotor Stage (Birth to age 2 years)

- Only the directive component is present at birth.
- The absence of myelination of the afferent pathways does not prevent transmission by the A-delta fibers.
- The development of body image is associated with specificity of the pain location, which is also dependent on the mother's response by pointing out where the child experienced the pain or trauma.
- Around 6 months, the child will focus on the area stimulated which results in visual attention, avoidance, and self-stimulation of the painful area.
- In young children, it is difficult to assess the cognitive component and its impact on the painful experience.

The Preoperational Stage (Age 2 to 7 years)

- Vocabulary expands but lacks abstraction.
- The child at this age views his world in concrete terms and is very self-centered.
- They do not trust the doctor or parents in exploring their pain or how to relieve it.
- At this stage the child has difficulty believing pain is beneficial and does not make a connection between pain and its cause.
- Children at this age tend to interpret pain as a form of punishment and they will have to be good to avoid future pain.
- At this age children will interpret diagnostics and treatment in the negative – this tendency to feel guilty decreases with age and is found more frequently in hospitalized children.

The Concrete Operational Stage (Age 8 to 10 years)

- Around this age children start to think in more abstract terms, but they do not understand the alarm value of pain.

- The child at this age can now understand the difference between internal and external events which helps them understand they may have come in contact with germs or have a disease.

- During this stage they have matured to a point where they accept directions from caregivers, even to accept painful treatments.

The Formal Operational Stage (Age 11 to 14 years)

- At this age children understand abstract thinking and can understand the causes of pain.
- Further, they can understand that the body can heal itself and are more aware of medical and psychological treatments.

Chronic Pain in Children

Next, we need to review in more depth the types of chronic pain children experience. The most frequent type of pain that children experience is headache, both tension and migraine. It is estimated that 20% of all pain in children is head pain, with migraine frequency increasing with age. Children with recurrent headache tend to be anxious, hypersensitive, and excessive worriers.[25] Recurrent headache also appears to run in families with at least one parent experiencing similar pain during their childhood.[29]

Abdominal pain is the second most frequent chronic pain in children. The incidence varies from 10% to 18% with the most frequent occurring between the ages of 8–10. There are several reasons forwarded to explain why this occurs. Children during this age tend to imitate their parents and if they see significant others reacting to stress in maladaptive ways, they will model similar coping styles. The research suggests that abdominal pain also tends to run in families where pain is a way of life.[25]

The third most frequent recurrent pain found in children is generally called limb or growing pain. This type of pain usually occurs between the ages of 8–12 and it affects about 4% to 15% of the children in this age range. It is difficult to treat since there is rarely any organic cause that can be determined and usually does not reflect any redness or swelling.[25]

Family Influences

The above research strongly suggests that most of the different types of recurrent pain that children experience are directly related to family influences, both genetic and environmental. When I evaluate a child who has recurrent pain, the inclusion of at least one parent or caregiver is required. If the child is appropriate for behavioral treatment, the parent is required to sit in and participate. If I teach the child relaxation techniques, the parent must also learn the same techniques. I have found this format useful, since they can practice together as a family in their own home. This approach is also beneficial since it reduces the pressure on the child as the identified patient and shifts the focus to the family.

Shifting the focus of treatment to the family has gained research support over the past decade. It is now recognized that parents who experience depression and anxiety have higher prevalence rates of children with chronic pain.[8] Further, the same research group found that mothers of children with functional abdominal pain were 4.9 times higher to have a history of depressive disorders and 4.8 times higher to have a history of anxiety disorders.

This pattern of familial influences on the incidence of pain appears to carry over into the adolescent years. Mothers of adolescents with pain exhibited more symptoms of stress, anxiety, and depression as compared to mothers with adolescents who were pain free.[14] Further, in a large population-based study in the Netherlands, maternal symptoms of anxiety during pregnancy predicted increased somatic complaints at 18 months of age.[49] We need to be careful not to over-interpret the research, which suggests that maternal mental health may predict or predispose a child to develop recurrent pain. Early identification of mothers at risk for mental health issues is improving and early intervention is becoming more proactive.

The role of dysfunctional cognitive issues with parents also appears to have influence on children who develop chronic pain.[36] As I mentioned in Chapter 4, the role of catastrophizing with adult pain patients also influences children who experience chronic pain. Research by Hechler, et al, suggested that mothers who demonstrated a high level of catastrophic thinking was related to the child's level of pain intensity.[19] Protective responses by parents have also been examined and the research suggests that frequently attending to pain symptoms including allowing the child to avoid regular activities is related to increased levels of disability in children with chronic pain.[13]

Pain Treatment with Children

The treatment of pain in children has changed dramatically in recent years, which is based on an accumulating body of research that indicates a more proactive approach is now warranted. In the past, children who experience recurrent pain were treated minimally or not at all. There were a number of factors that contributed to this mindset including the fear of addiction, a lack of knowledge on how children communicate, and limited information regarding pediatric anesthesia.[7, 39]

First, any treatment plan involving children should be based on a multidisciplinary approach. Keep in mind the main difference between the child and the adult patient is that the child is usually fearful, which requires pain providers to be patient, supportive, and understanding. Adult patients have a greater knowledge base that mitigates fear and misunderstanding for the most part. Providers should also be familiar with child development, physically, emotionally, and mentally. Family related influences must be taken into account as they may contribute to making the pain worse. Often children are overlooked when the pain provider is explaining the treatment. The child needs to be included by presenting the treatment in terms they can understand and reassured that the treatment will be helpful.

Finally, it is important to include the parents or caregiver in this process, since the child will look to them for emotional support.[29]

Physical Approaches to Treatment

Surgical and anesthetic techniques are rarely used with children, but can play a role in exceptional cases. Pain providers who employ these techniques need to possess special skills that include a caring and sensitive bedside manner.

The use of massage and therapeutic touch has been found useful to providers who have experience in working with children. It is also helpful to teach parents these techniques so that they can provide additional emotional and physical support when providers are not available. Parents and providers should realize that children are more sensitive to physical contact as compared to adults.

The use of acupuncture is rarely used because of the fear of needles in children, although there is one study on the use of acupuncture in a pediatric population that reported a high level of success.[23] Additionally, there is another study supporting the use of TENS in a pediatric sample that demonstrated positive effects.[29] Physical and occupational therapies appear indicated since they are consistent with a child's need for movement and activity. This approach could include the use of stretching, especially if the parent can model the activity and make it fun.

Behavioral Approaches

In my own practice, I have used relaxation therapy augmented by biofeedback with both children and adolescents. The youngest child I have treated was a girl, age 8, who presented with recurrent headaches. I remember that she was exceptionally curious which helped her understand the nature of her pain. I should also mention that her mother sat in and also learned the same techniques so that they could practice together in their own home. She and her mom both did well and the frequency and intensity of her headache pain subsided to a point where all pain medicines were discontinued.

The inclusion of parent participation is helpful since it assists with generalization in the child's environment, especially in identifying triggers that may be a result of a painful episode. Adolescents present a unique challenge since sometimes they do not want their parents present. If that is the case, I will meet with the parents separately to go over treatment goals and approaches.

The research support for cognitive-based behavioral therapy with children has expanded in recent years. Initially this support focused on children who presented with recurrent headache.[43] Research has expanded to include abdominal, musculoskeletal, and disease-related pain.[33] Research support for the inclusion of parent strategies is growing, according to Palermo, which included the use of operant learning techniques. The focus of this approach is modifying parents' response to pain complaints and encouraging adaptive methods to promote well-being.[33]

In a related recent systematic review of parent interventions for chronic health conditions, by the same research group, it was found that problem solving therapy was helpful in improving parent mental health.[33]

Pain in Older Adults

The assessment and treatment of recurrent pain with older adults, as with children, present special challenges for the health care provider. Over the course of thirty years of practice, I have assessed and treated a fair number of older adult pain patients.

On a personal note, I am now in the category of an "older adult" who lives with recurrent pain on a daily basis. Not that this experience gives me any special insight, but I do practice what I preach. In hindsight, my experience as a pain psychologist has taught me not to over-generalize or group older adults as being the same just because they are older. On the contrary, I have found considerable variation across the entire older pain patient population. Each patient presents with unique coping skills, history, and intellectual skills that need to be considered when evaluating and treating the older adult with recurrent pain.

Numbers and Pain Types

The growth of research studies focusing on the older adult has increased considerably over the past two decades. This growth can be explained, in part, due to the growing numbers of older adults over the age of 65 who currently make up approximately 10% of the total population and by 2030 will represent 20%.[26] According to the Administration on Aging, older adults are the fastest growing segment of the population with an average of 10,000 individuals turning 65 every day, with a projected population of 72 million older adults living in the United States by 2030, according to the US Census Bureau.[10]

Further, according to the Centers for Disease Control and Prevention, over two-thirds of older Americans suffer from multiple chronic conditions and treatment for these conditions comprise 66% of the total health care budget.[10] It is estimated that 60–75% of people over 65, report persistent pain.[44]

The specific breakdown of pain types within the older population are:[17]

65%	osteoarthritic back and neck pain
40%	musculoskeletal pain
35%	peripheral neuropathic pain (due to diabetes or post-therapeutic neuralgia)
15–25%	chronic joint pain

Tsang found that the prevalence of pain increases with age and women are more likely to report persistent pain as compared to men.[44] In a European survey, Langley found that most older adults describe their pain as moderate (60%) and 25% describe it as severe.[24]

Exercise and the Older Adult

Chronic pain in the older population has a widespread impact on a variety of problems including activity restriction, sleep issues, and mood, to name a few. Limiting activity due to pain is a natural instinctual response, but in the case of persistent pain, it becomes a counterproductive strategy that can lead to more pain.[22, 47] In my own practice, finding an appropriate activity for every patient is a primary goal in the treatment plan.

The older patient presents a unique challenge in finding an activity they feel comfortable performing. Usually the largest hurdle to overcome is the fear of falling. Often, older people reduce their activity level and gain weight, compromising their flexibility which increases the fear of falling.[40] Weight gain also places more stress on the knees, hips, and back, and often results in more pain.[28]

Besides walking, the one activity I strongly recommend to my patients is warm water exercise. This form of activity removes the fear of falling and if the patient is overweight, it reduces the stress on joints since they are weightless. Usually I recommend they start by walking in the pool in waist-deep water, working up to deeper levels, which increases resistance and builds strength. Once they achieve a level of comfort and increased strength, they can graduate to wearing a flotation belt, which allows them to walk or jog in deeper water. Eventually, they can work up to a water exercise class designed for older adults, which provides the additional benefit of group support. The class I attend spends at least 10 minutes before and after the class devoted to stretching in the water. The chief advantage of warm water is that it relaxes the muscles, which promotes a greater stretch. The pool I use maintains a water temperature around 90°F, which I find about perfect. For the more severely impaired patient, physical therapy in a warm pool is advised and it is usually covered under most insurance plans with a physician's order.

Pain and Sleep in the Older Adult

In the previous chapter I discussed the relationship between pain and sleep, but the older patient presents additional challenges. Older patients with persistent pain are twice as likely to report sleep problems that include sleep onset delay and excessive time in bed.[11] According to Valentine, et al, 42% of middle-aged and older patients with persistent pain experience chronic sleep deprivation that contributes to more inactivity and subsequent daytime fatigue.[45]

Further, as I pointed out in the chapter on sleep and pain, older adults produce less melatonin, which influences the regulation of sleep cycles. It is generally believed by sleep medicine specialists that lower melatonin levels in older adults is a major factor why adults over 70 usually sleep less.[32]

I always consult with the patient's referring physician before recommending adjunctive melatonin as a sleep aid. Keep in mind that melatonin has a relatively short half-life, therefore it will only be effective in helping the patient initiate sleep. There are extended release formulations available in both pill and sublingual preparations.

Behavioral Therapy with Older Adults

Behavioral therapy techniques are appropriate for the older adult provided they are not confused or that their memory is not compromised. I have found in my own practice that relaxation techniques can be effective if the patient is carefully selected. I will also add temperature biofeedback to augment relaxation procedures. Please refer to the chapter on treatment for a more in-depth discussion. I remember one 85 year-old patient who was still actively farming who was coping with moderate levels of persistent pain and a significant sleep problem. It is important to note that he was a highly motivated individual who was open to new experiences. He could not get enough relaxation therapy, always wanting more to achieve a deeper state of relaxation. When he felt more in control of his pain, his sleep improved, and these were powerful reinforcements. Another factor to consider with the older adult is a propensity to worry, which results in a higher level of psycho-physiological arousal. If your patient is cold in the extremities with possible color changes, temperature biofeedback may be indicated.

Mood Issues with the Older Adult

As I mentioned in both Chapters 2 and 3, a majority of chronic pain patients are at risk for depression. The incidence of severe depression in the older adult with persistent pain ranges from 19–28%.[18] Even though this association appears significant, not all older pain patients are depressed. A study by Corran reported that 75% of older adult pain patients who were being treated in a multidisciplinary pain clinic reported reasonable levels of pain control and low levels of depression.[16]

I have found in my own practice that many older adult patients, both men and women, generally understate their symptoms. This stoic presentation should be considered when assessing the older pain patient, since it is easy to overlook a major mood issue. When I discuss pain and depression with my older patients, I will use the metaphor of a horse and buggy; what one does the other will follow. Chou discussed this reciprocal relationship between pain and depression in the older adult with pain predicting increases in depression and depression predicting increases in pain.[12]

Unfortunately, access to mental health care for older adults with pain is difficult, especially in rural areas. Szczerbinska, et al, found that in almost one half of their sample of older adults, mental health undertreatment increases with age in home care and institutional settings.[42]

Physical Changes and the Perception of Pain

Physical changes in the older adult can influence the perception of pain. Recent research findings now confirm that aging is associated with changes in the structure, function, and chemistry of the nervous system that directly impact the perception of pain. One example of change pointed out by Dr. Antonio Verdu Mestre, et al, is that the density of unmyelinated fibers in the peripheral nervous system decreases with age.[46]

This reduction in density will also result in a slowing of nerve conduction. The changes we see with aging are a complex process that is not well understood. Recent evidence suggests that older adults are unique regarding their perception of pain.

As I mentioned earlier, older adults tend to downplay pain symptoms as compared to other chronic medical conditions. Keep in mind that this generation experienced a world war and a major economic depression. In my opinion, those experiences had a profound influence on these individuals in coping with adversity; it was not socially accepted to talk about or admit you lived with pain. In addition, there is evidence to suggest that the acceptance of pain as "age normative" may act as a psychological buffer or protective mechanism to counteract the emotional reactivity associated with the pain experience.[48] It is important for all health care providers to be aware of this behavior of the older individual in understating their pain. Further, it is equally important for the health care provider not to dismiss the importance of multidisciplinary pain management for the older adult with recurrent pain.

Social Support and the Perception of Pain

The role of social support is just as important for the older adult as it is for the younger adult in coping with chronic pain. In the older adult, social support is different in form and function since they report fewer friends and social supports as compared to younger adults.[21]

Further, the feeling among older adults is that emotional well-being is associated with a few close friends as compared to many friends or a broad social support network. This reduction in the size of one's social support network may be due, in part, to the amount of energy expended in maintaining a large network of friends. In addition, as we age we tend to be more selective in our friendships. In some cases, social support is critical for the older adult who experiences persistent pain. As we age, we rely on others to help with activities of daily living, transportation, and monitoring health issues, including medicine.

The Role of Medicine with the Older Adult

As we age, we also rely more on medicine to maintain a quality of life both in prescription form and over the counter supplements. Recent research indicates that older adults take between 5–8 daily medicines with 12–39% taking more than 9.[9] These numbers will likely grow as the older population becomes larger due to the baby boom generation.

The use of OTC (over the counter) preparations has also escalated in the older population. Adults over the age of 65 represent about 12% of the population and use 40% of all over the counter preparations.[37] This trend in self-medicating can be potentially problematic for the older adult who is coping with chronic pain. Adverse drug interactions among the older population are on the rise with some estimates reaching 20%.[38]

As we age physically, our ability to process medicines also changes. I will outline a few of these changes. For those of you who want a more in-depth discussion, the review by Wooten published in 2012 is an excellent resource.[50]

According to this review, aging is associated with reduced drug absorption due to reduced gastrointestinal motility and blood flow. Further, there are changes in muscle mass and an increase in body fat, poorer drug metabolism due to decreases in hepatic blood flow and liver mass, and reduced excretion due to declines in renal function. There is also evidence to suggest that molecular changes with aging may be associated with receptor sensitivity to certain drug classes.[31]

For the older adult who experiences multiple health issues, including pain, the implications for negative health outcomes are considerable. Therefore, I always advise my older patients to work closely with their primary care physicians in regulating their medications, including the use of over the counter preparations. Recently, I have found that pharmacists are more accommodating in researching potential adverse drug interactions. For more information on this important topic I would refer the reader to the *American Geriatric Society Panel on the Pharmacological Management of Persistent Pain in Older Adults* published in 2009.[1]

Cognitive Issues with the Older Patient

The influence of memory loss or dementia is an important consideration when treating the older adult who lives with persistent pain. According to Corbett, et al, it appears that 30–50% of older adults diagnosed with dementia experience persistent pain.[15] When you combine dementia and pain a number of behaviors can occur including aggression, agitation, and confusion. Further, a popular misconception that older adults with dementia feel and experience less pain may contribute to an underassessment and under treatment of pain.[27] The consensus of research suggests that older adults with dementia experience pain differently but the perception of pain severity does not change.[6]

Summary

To conclude this section on pain in the older adult, my own personal experience tells me that this population presents a special challenge for many reasons. This generation of older adults has experienced many hardships including a world war and a major economic depression. These hardships have contributed to a mindset of stoicism (being brave in the face of pain). This mindset of stoicism presents a number of challenges to the health care provider. Do you overlook the possibility the older adult may be experiencing greater psychosocial distress but deny any discomfort? How can the provider penetrate this shield of defense when standard health care practice limits the primary care physician to an average of 11 minutes per visit. With the older adult, trust is an important influence that takes time to build. Trust helps reduce fear, which I feel explains, in part, this shield of being brave. If the primary care physician suspects that the older adult patient is understating their pain symptoms, they should refer the patient to a multidisciplinary pain program. The primary basis for this referral is that you need time and a variety of providers to fully evaluate the existence of a serious pain issue. If the older adult is understating their pain, it may result in a number of related mental health issues, especially depression. Therefore, it is incumbent upon the health care provider to assess for comorbid conditions. I realize there is much wisdom in the old adage of "letting sleeping dogs lie," but do not overlook the older patient who is reaching out for help.

7 Gender and Pain

Equality consists in the same treatment of similar persons.
–Aristotle

Introduction

THE MAIN FOCUS OF THIS CHAPTER IS TO EXPLORE THE QUESTION: Do men and women perceive and react to pain differently? And do men and women use different coping strategies when they experience recurrent or chronic pain? These questions are relevant to pain providers when assessing and developing treatment plans for patients who experience and live with pain on a daily basis.

Twenty-five years ago, when I was on the faculty at Oregon Health Sciences University (OHSU), one of our medical psychology residents came to me for advice. She was looking for a research topic she could explore during her residency. I suggested she consider the issue of gender differences in relation to the pain experience. At that time, very little was known about this topic so I encouraged her to review the research that was available. She also consulted with other faculty members about the advisability of exploring this topic, and after careful deliberation, she decided that the topic of gender and pain was too politically sensitive. Naturally, I was disappointed in her decision, but I understood her reluctance to pursue a controversial research project in a conservative medical school environment.

The topic of gender and pain is more accepted today as shown by the recent growth in the body of research literature. It is now accepted that men and women do experience pain differently. There are a number of promising research approaches attempting to address the causes of these differences. I will review these new areas of research that will help us to understand the role of gender as it applies to the pain experience.

A major review of the research on gender and pain published in 1995 confirmed recent findings that women do experience more pain compared to men.[25] This review suggested that women have a lower pain threshold and tolerance to experimental pain that included mechanical, thermal, and electrical stimuli.[33] The 1995 review pointed out a number of issues when comparing men and women that contribute to the variability between the two genders.

Dao and LeResche listed a number of factors[11] that contribute to this variability including:

- Dimensions of pain measured
- Type of stimulus
- Characteristics of the experimental environment

- Spatial aspects of the stimulus
- Characteristics of the subject
- Temporal aspects of the stimulus

I believe an additional factor must be controlled, and that is the sex of the experimenter. It is well understood that both men and women react differently to the demand characteristics of the experimenter and whether the experimenter is a male or a female.

A well-designed study by Fillingin, et al, stated that sex differences in response to pain is well documented but the mechanisms underlying these differences are not well understood.[17] Fillingin proposed that gender roles and pain responses could be mediated by perceived ability to tolerate pain. In other words, stereotypic sex roles are perceived to influence greater tolerance for pain between men than women. The results of this study indicated men showing higher pain tolerance but also higher blood pressure (BP) responses. Fillingin pointed out that a body of evidence suggested higher resting BP is associated with lower pain sensitivity. One interesting explanation forwarded by the authors was that men tried harder to tolerate the pain resulting in higher systolic blood pressure (SBP). Also keep in mind that (SBP) is related to sympathetic arousal. The authors concluded that perceived ability to tolerate pain may have influenced the relationship between cardiovascular variables and pain tolerance.[15]

In a related study by Frot, men revealed a significant positive correlation between anxiety (sympathetic arousal) and pain intensity, and women did not.[18] The results of this study support the general conclusion that women perceive experimental pain as more intense compared to men. The results also support the findings of Fillingin that gender differences in pain perception may be related to a strong C-fiber component, and the idea that men are more bothered or upset by chronic pain compared to women.

A meta-analytic study by Riley, et al, reviewed research using experimentally-induced pain that provided evidence of the magnitude of gender differences in pain.[33] This study pointed out a number of assumptions relevant to gender differences, including cultural and physiological influences. For example, males have been socialized to suppress outward signs of pain. Riley, et al, also mentioned the important influence of the menstrual cycle on pain perception. Females demonstrated more pain sensitivity following a mid-cycle surge during the luteal phase.[33]

Sarlani, et al, conducted an interesting study examining the concept of temporal summation as it relates to gender and pain. Temporal summation of pain is the increase in pain intensity after repetitive noxious stimulation of constant intensity. Temporal summation is regarded as a psycho-physiological correlate of wind-up. As we discussed in The Nature of Pain, wind-up is the increase in the magnitude of second order nociceptive neuron responses when repetitive noxious stimuli of constant strength are applied. The authors believe that wind-up and temporal summation of pain share common features and have a central basis. Current thinking suggests that temporal summation in women is upregulated at a greater rate than men. Results of this study suggested that women may be more easily upregulated into pathological hyper-excitability which accounts for a higher prevalence of various pain conditions.[38]

Pain Medicine and Gender

The fact that men and women respond differently to pain medicine is an important issue in the practice of pain management. The most frequently prescribed pain medicines belong in the opioid class. As I mentioned in Chapter 4, opioids work through specific opioid receptors that are well documented. Three types of opioid receptors have been identified: mu, delta, and kappa, with mu and kappa the most frequent in humans.[25] Research by Craft found that women use 40% less opioid-based medicine than men for postoperative pain.[9] This finding was confirmed by research conducted by Miaskowski, et al.[27]

There are several factors that could explain the differential response to pain medicine between men and women. First, we know that sex hormones can modulate the density of opioid receptors.[22] Additionally, research on sex hormones indicates improved mu receptor binding in some brain regions in women as measured by PET scans.[30, 42] Further, recent advances in genetics have revealed greater opioid analgesia in women for specific receptor genes that mediate female responses.[27]

Finally, it is important to remember that psychological factors also influence the response to opioid-based therapy. Anxiety or sympathetic reactivity imposes a major negative influence in pain perception and brain activity.[20]

Biological Factors that Influence the Perception of Pain

In 2000, Roger Fillingin published a bio-psychosocial model that has influenced the thinking about the differences between genders that is evident today. The factors he proposed that are responsible for the differences are:

- Biological factors that included sex hormones and endogenous pain control mechanisms

- Psychological factors that include anxiety and negative affect, and

- Sociocultural factors that include gender role expectations of pain.

The model also shows that the perception of pain is influenced by the interaction of all these factors working together in a relative fashion.[15] For those of you who are interested in this topic, I would highly recommend a volume by Fillingin published by the IASP press.[16]

Sex hormones, according to this model, are relevant to the evaluation and treatment of pain.[24] When considering all of the biological factors, the role of sex hormones has received the most research attention. According to Marchand, sex hormones in the central nervous system (CNS) have been documented to influence the neurotransmitters that are involved in the perception of pain.[25]

In a recent well-designed study, it was demonstrated that changes in the plasma level of estrogen influenced changes in serotonin, acetylcholine, dopamine, and endorphins.[1] Additional research examined the role of progesterone and found similar influences on levels of dopamine and acetylcholine.[27] The main sex hormones in women are estrogen and progesterone, which will vary according to the menstrual cycle. It should be noted that testosterone is also present in women but 10 to

15 times less as compared to men. Further, girls and boys react to pain in a similar fashion before puberty but differently after puberty, which tends to fade when levels of sex hormones decrease.[36]

Estrogen receptors have been found in the dorsal horn, which suggests mechanisms that could regulate pain sensitivity by influencing neurotransmitters, including Substance P, GABA, dopamine, serotonin and norepinephrine.[2] One of the conclusions forwarded from this research is that a decrease in estrogen would increase sensitivity to pain. Conversely, an increase in estrogen would promote an analgesic effect by stimulating a bolus of inhibiting transmitters.[2]

It appears that testosterone plays a protective role in decreasing the perception of pain.[19] An example of this protective role was suggested recently in a study investigating the protective effect testosterone plays in rheumatoid arthritis (RA), which affects three times as many women as men.[37] Further evidence was demonstrated when men who experience RA reported fewer affected joints after taking testosterone.[10]

Psychosocial Influences

Fillingin's model included the importance of psychosocial influences that contribute to why men and women respond differently to pain. One question that is frequently raised is the weight given to each factor in Fillingin's model, biological and psychosocial.[16] In my opinion, Fillingin's biosocial model would answer that it is a reciprocal interaction between the two factors. To determine the amount of weight given to each factor is a difficult task since it is a dynamic model that will change depending on the internal and external forces that are in play at any given moment.

Anxiety at a clinical level includes both cognitive and physiological contributions that have an accumulative impact on the perception of pain and how we cope with that perception. As an emotional state, anxiety can be described as hyper-vigilant tension that is usually associated with the unpleasant feeling of fear.[31]

The psycho-physiological component of anxiety is reflected in an elevated sympathetic nervous system reaction. It is well accepted that elevated levels of anxiety increases the perception of pain.[39] This finding is independent of the intensity of the painful stimulus. Recent research looks at the influence of anxiety in relation to gender differences and the reaction to pain. Both clinical and experimental studies have found that increased pain sensitivity was associated with anxiety in men but not women.[18, 20, 13, 32]

It is important to point out that, historically, the concept of anxiety was divided into two categories: State and Trait Anxiety. State Anxiety implies a time-limited state, or "an anxious state," as compared to Trait Anxiety, which is a longer lasting or a more permanent feature of the personality. One study suggested that men feel more State Anxiety associated with pain or that a man's reaction (anxiety) is more time-limited as compared to women.[32] Another study on the topic suggested that women may have a lower level of State Anxiety as it relates to pain but a higher level of Trait Anxiety independent of pain.[20]

The anxiety differences between men and women have been examined from experimental pain research. In men, acute stress and State Anxiety is associated with increased opioid inhibitory response and higher levels of cortisol.[6, 30] This finding may help explain gender differences by suggesting that men, when they experience elevated levels of State Anxiety, also activate descending inhibitory mechanisms. The important point to remember is that any anxiety, State or Trait, will increase the perception of pain. The differences between men and women may be explained by dividing anxiety into the two separate factors. State Anxiety is related to pain perception in men and Trait Anxiety in women.[20]

The role of depression and gender has also been examined extensively in recent years. The overall evidence suggests that depression is a significant predictor for the development of chronic pain.[7] Further, the research supports the finding that as the number of depressive symptoms increase, the result will be more pain.[4] The prevalence of depression in patients who experience chronic pain suggests a wide range from a low of 30% to a high of 54% of the total pain population.[3] The question that must be answered is, does depression influence the role of pain between the genders?

The research would suggest that an association exists between depressive symptoms and increased somatic focus only for women.[5] Somatic focus influences the report of pain and the consensus of research suggests that depression is positively correlated with pain in women and not men.[21, 26] As mentioned earlier, Marchand pointed out that depression is related to reduced opioid analgesia. He proposes that this link could explain, in part, why women perceive more pain than men.[25]

Anger and Pain

It is well understood that negative emotions, such as anger, magnify the pain experience.[35] We also now know that pain does not generate the same emotional response across both genders. The research would suggest that women become more frustrated and men become more anxious when coping with persistent pain.[34] Specifically, anger is associated with greater sensitivity to acute pain and more intensity to persistent pain.[17] Conversely, it is interesting to note that positive emotions inhibit the pain response and facilitate coping.[32]

I remember reading Norman Cousins' *Anatomy of an Illness,* which was published in 1979. At that time he was experiencing a serious collagen illness – a disease of the connective tissue. He talked about the work of Walter B. Cannon who introduced the concept of homeostatic responses, or natural processes that enable the individual to return to the "normal" state before it experienced the noxious influence. He also referenced the work of William Osler, who felt that successful healing was due to the individual's personality and behavior independent of medicine. So in cooperation with his doctors, he developed a program to enhance positive affirmative emotions with the goal of enhancing body chemistry. In order to achieve this goal he used funny movies such as Marx Brothers' films to generate genuine belly laughter. The program worked, inflammation was reduced and he experienced more pain-free sleep. I still recommend this book to patients and the feedback is usually positive.[8]

Cognition and Pain

How we think about pain and the language we use to describe our pain are very important cognitive factors that ultimately influence how we react and cope with persistent pain. The research today would suggest that women use more emotional and social strategies to cope with pain, while men use more active approaches to problem solving.[41]

In my opinion, the explanation for this difference is based in how boys and girls are socialized. This opinion is based on a well-designed study conducted in the 1960s where Mechanic found that boys express their pain less than girls.[27] It has been suggested that masculine behavior is more narrowly-defined and rigid compared to feminine behavior. As I mentioned earlier, a family history of pain has a more profound influence on women than men.[16]

In a related recent study, it was suggested that young girls express more emotional distress when they experience pain as compared to boys. This same study indicated that girls are more adept at using social and emotional support from those around them compared to boys.[14]

The role of catastrophizing in recent years has become a major predictive factor in outcome studies involving pain treatment. Edwards, et al, designed a study examining catastrophizing as a mediator of gender differences in both recurrent daily pain and experimental pain.[12]

The results of this study suggested that gender differences in recurrent daily pain are due to levels of catastrophizing. However, the results did not support the higher threshold and tolerance levels in thermal and cold pain observed in men. The authors stated that catastrophizing appears to emerge relatively early in development and is more common among adolescent girls.

A well-designed study by Keefe, et al, examined the role of gender differences with pain coping and mood in individuals with osteoarthritic knee pain. What was unique about this study is the format of multiple pain ratings twice a day (afternoon and evening) for 30 days.[23] The results indicated that women used more problem-focused coping compared to men. Women who catastrophized were less likely to report negative mood. Considering pain ratings across the day, women exhibited an increase in pain over the course of the day. Men exhibited an increase in coping efficacy over the day. Finally, men experienced more negative mood in the morning after an evening of increased pain. The uniqueness of this study pointed out the importance of obtaining multiple daily assessments when studying gender differences.[23]

Gender and Neurological Differences

Research examining neural differences between the genders when presented with a painful stimulus has gained more attention in recent years. Improvements in brain imaging have provided additional information that helps us understand how men and women respond to pain. A Canadian research group, using healthy normal subjects, found a positive relationship in activation differences between men and women.[40] Their findings suggested that women, not men, demonstrate a strong positive linear relationship between perigenual anterior cingulated cortex (pg ACC) and the report of pain. This finding is consistent with other research suggesting that women are more emotionally responsive and perceptive when presented with a negative emotional experience. Tremblay, et al, suggested that men deactivate prefrontal suppression when processing pain, which leads to the mobilization of threat control circuits when experiencing pain.

What evolutionary purpose could explain gender differences in relation to the pain experience? Tremblay, et al, has speculated that over time, men have occupied the role of hunter and defender against aggressive behavior so they have learned to cope with pain in order to survive, compared to women, who have developed a strong sense of trust and sensitivity, which promotes strong social bonds that supports survival of the group.[40]

Conclusion

Writing this chapter presented a number of challenges that motivated me to present a fair and balanced analysis of this topic. As a scientific community, pain medicine and pain management has evolved and matured since I started practicing some thirty years ago. During this time, new technology has helped us understand the importance of how gender can impact the pain experience.

I hope all pain providers incorporate these findings to improve treatment plans that will ultimately benefit all patients coping with persistent pain.

Chapter

8 Pain and Surgery

Psychological Factors That May Influence Elective Surgical Outcomes

QUESTIONNAIRES SUCH AS Minnesota Multiphasic Personality Inventory (MMPI) and McGill Pain Questionnaire (MPS), as well as psychological examination, may help determine which chronic pain patients will have successful surgical outcomes or not.

Elective Surgery for Pain Relief

Pain relief is the primary reason why patients undergo elective surgery in the United States. This chapter will attempt to point out a number of psychological factors that should be considered before elective surgery is considered in patients experiencing persistent or chronic pain. To determine the best candidates for surgery, clinicians should evaluate each patient individually, taking into consideration the extensiveness of the procedure and the patient's degree of motivation in their rehabilitation.

Thirty years ago, when I became interested in pain management, I reviewed the pain literature in depth. I was looking for a framework or model from which to evaluate and treat chronic pain patients. At that time I was also interested in psychophysiology and biofeedback, which I felt was complimentary to my interest in pain management. The Gate Control Model of Pain, introduced by Ron Melzack, PhD, and Patrick Wall, MA, DM, in 1965, appealed to me since it was based on credible, empirical evidence, and it has practical face value. Since the 1960s, psychological approaches to chronic pain have been greatly influenced by their work.

The Gate Control Model offered a legitimate alternative to the dualistic approach (either psychogenic or "real" notion) to chronic pain. Since its publication, there have been over 2,000 published peer-reviewed studies based on the Gate Control Model. Both Patrick Wall (now deceased) and Ron Melzack have updated the original model.

Factors Influencing Pain Perception

Melzack, et al, believed there are three primary interdependent factors that influence pain: the sensory factor, the affective factor (or how we cope with chronic pain), and the evaluative/cognitive factor (or how we think about our pain). When I evaluate a pain patient who is being considered for elective surgery, my clinical impressions are based on Melzack's model.

Although most of my colleagues in pain management are very knowledgeable about the sensory influence in pain, what they may not appreciate is how the affective and cognitive factors influence the pain signal. Pain is a perception and if you want to be successful in your treatment you need to treat the perception. In other words, you may perform an excellent surgery or intervention, but patients who are depressed, constant worriers, or magnifying their symptoms, may inform you six months down the road that their pain is worse.

Patient Examination

Most of my pain referrals are not overly receptive about being evaluated by a pain psychologist due to the misperception that the psychologist's role is to determine if the patient's pain is real or imaginary. This stereotype is based on outdated, invalid, dualistic assumptions about the either/or nature of pain.

When I initially meet pain patients, I attempt to defuse the either/or notion by drawing a Venn diagram of three interlocking circles. I inform the patients that my job is to assist the referring physician in understanding the affective and/or cognitive factors that may be influencing their pain, not to question the validity of whether their pain is real. Initially, I draw the circles with identical sizes. After the evaluation, I sit down with the patient and redraw the Venn diagram based on my clinical impression. I point out the interrelated nature of pain and how these factors contribute to their pain experience and form the basis of a treatment plan.

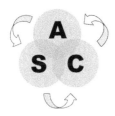

In this illustration, the darkest shaded area in the very center is pain. The affective and cognitive factors are contributory, especially if the patient is depressed and is exhibiting catastrophic thinking. This is not a stimulus-response linear model, but a circular, interdependent and reciprocal process that is very dynamic. Mood and thinking can change from day to day, which contributes to pain levels being very labile. A point to always keep in mind is that all pain patients are unique, which presents certain challenges to the pain specialist not to over generalize or think that all pain patients are the same.

Another important cognitive risk factor is how the patients think about their pain. Is the pain troublesome or is it killing them? The difference between these two descriptive adjectives is clinically significant. I first started to appreciate the clinical significance of catastrophic thinking after reading a study conducted by Wilbert E. Fordyce and Stanley Bigos, in 1992. It was an extensive and well-designed study where over 3,000 Boeing employees were administered the MMPI. The sample was then followed for three years to determine if a profile could predict who would file a back injury claim. An elevated Scale 3 appeared to be a significant predictor of subsequent back injury. In my opinion, Scale 3 is a good indicator of catastrophic thinking or what I refer to as the "Chicken Little factor."

While at OHSU I conducted a study to determine if we could predict, based on a psychological profile, who would fail a trial of spinal cord stimulation.[1, 2, 3] Scale 3 of the MMPI was found to be a significant predictor of trial failure. These patients with catastrophic thinking are easy to identify just by asking them to describe their pain, or by administering the McGill Pain Questionnaire (MPS) with particular attention to group 16. Melzack constructed the MPS based on his model of pain. I would strongly recommend to the reader his book Pain Measurement and Assessment for a more detailed explanation.

Further evidence of catastrophic thinking can be obtained by asking the patient to rate their pain on a 0–10 point scale, with 10 being the highest rating. The catastrophic pain patient will usually rate their pain at a 10 or higher, even knowing that the scale only goes to 10, and will also describe very little variability over the course of a day. These patients will typically present themselves in a dramatic fashion, usually magnifying their symptoms, which will not be consistent with physical findings. In addition, they will usually be more antalgic and hyper-responsive to physical testing. If you perform physiological testing, they will generally be colder in the extremities, have elevated sweat gland activity (EDR or GRS), and exhibit higher surface muscle activity (EMG) readings. In the extreme, these patients may be diagnosed with some type of anxiety disorder or elevated psychophysiologic sympathetic arousal.

The surgeon who is considering an elective procedure on a pain patient who is consistent with this typology should proceed with caution. The prudent course of action would include a psychological evaluation from a pain psychologist before proceeding with any major invasive procedure.

Caveats to MMPI Questionnaire

There is a caveat regarding the use of the MMPI with any chronic illness patient, including pain. The MMPI and its newer versions are the most frequently utilized psychological tests in the medical setting. However, they are also often misused, especially if the physician relies on a canned actuarial computer-generated report. Actuarial interpretations are based on cutoff scores that may distort interpretations because of construct validity issues. Over the course of my career, I have administered over 5,000 MMPIs to chronic pain patients. Because of the way the questions are constructed, especially on Scale 1, the typical pain patient will score high, triggering a canned interpretation of conversion. If the clinician reading the report is not aware of this issue, it will lead to a false interpretation. Additionally, this report becomes part of the patient's permanent medical record and this distortion is then perpetuated into the future with profound negative consequences. As a cognitively-based pain psychologist, I interpret elevated Scale 1 scores as predictable considering the form of the questions, and this becomes part of the patient's treatment plan. The MMPI can be a useful tool if used properly by an experienced pain psychologist.

Expectations of Surgery

An additional cognitive issue that is often overlooked in the presurgical evaluation is the patient's expectation of the surgery outcome. The patient's expectation is clinically significant and should not be discounted, especially if patients expect their pain to disappear. We are creatures of a fix-it culture: if it is broken, let's fix it. This typology usually describes a concrete, rigid thinker. It's black or white; there are no shades of grey. Further, based on my experience, I suspect that this substantial subset of patients who exhibit a cognitive mindset that includes catastrophic thinking and unrealistic expectations, contributes, in part, to a placebo response. This is especially relevant when considering implantable pain technology. The patient may report a successful trial and then six months down the road it stops working and the patient wants it removed. This explanation results in the worst case scenario, which contributes to doubt, not only by the implanting physician, but also by the insurance company who underwrote the procedure.

From a cognitive-behavioral perspective I explain to the patient that surgery and or implantable pain technology is only one tool that is added to the patient's pain management tool box. The more tools the patient has in their pain management tool box, the better able they are to manage their pain. The cognitive therapeutic premise is that the patient accepts the fact that it is their pain; they own it and therefore it is their responsibility to manage it as best they can. Further, these tools, including pharmaceutical, implantable, and behavioral, are not mutually exclusive but should be considered complimentary and additive.

Algorithm

Finally, I would like to propose a theoretical model that continues to be a work in progress. My goal is to offer a pragmatic algorithm that assists the pain management specialist with patients who present with complex psychosocial symptoms. Referring patients for surgery is a very personal process that is greatly influenced by experience, training, and individual temperament. Any decision-making algorithm has to keep this individuality in place, and I believe the following model achieves that goal.

I would encourage each practitioner to list all the psychosocial factors that are relevant to them and give them a weighted score. For example, a serious mood disorder would be weighted higher than a milder mood disorder. Further, keep in mind that the vertical axis is additive.

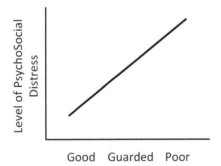

Conclusion

The psychosocial factors discussed in this chapter are not exhaustive and each surgeon can add other factors that they feel are important in their decision-making process. For example, in this chapter, I did not include such factors as mood, addiction or drug abuse, confusion or memory problems, age, and sleep disorders. I am hopeful that the above model gives the individual surgeon a framework to formulate decisions that will promote and contribute to improved patient outcome and welfare.

Recently, I was asked by the State of Oregon Workers' Compensation Division to evaluate a patient who had undergone 12 back surgeries. His neurosurgeon, who had performed all of his previous surgeries, now recommended number thirteen. The patient wanted his back fixed and he would not consider implantable pain options. The patient was very rigid in his thinking, which in his case was counterproductive, since he expected to be pain free. This patient exhibited a number of cognitive and affective risk factors that contributed to a poor outcome prognosis. First, he engaged in superstitious or magical thinking. Second, he was suspicious of having a mechanical device inside his body. Finally, he was a very angry individual, which is considered an affective risk factor. Anger contributes to a constant state of sympathetic reactivity which has a direct influence on pain perception.

Chapter

9 Motivation and Trust

Building Trust with Unmotivated Patients

MOTIVATION IS CRITICAL TO THE OUTCOME for the pain patient. If they experience unsuccessful medical or surgical treatments, they become discouraged and resist further treatment. If the pain professionals are not involved early in the treatment process, they must approach the patient with a set of strategies for building trust.

The referral process is an important component to understand, not only from the patient perspective, but also from the provider viewpoint. This initial step in the process usually starts with the primary care physician (PCP). A History and Physical evaluation and a preliminary diagnosis by the PCP starts the ball rolling and influences the direction or path the patient will follow. The primary physician may treat the patient's pain initially, which can also include adjunctive supportive care. The numbers are impressive. According to a recent report by the Institute of Medicine (IOM) entitled *Relieving Pain in America* chronic pain conditions affect at least 116 million adults at a cost of $560–635 billion annually in direct medical treatment costs and lost productivity.[4]

How many of that 116 million could be classified as difficult or unmotivated patients? That depends on a number of factors. Some patients start the process with existing emotional issues, such as anger, anxiety, or depression, which may predispose the patient to transition from acute to chronic pain. Based on my experience, the process of the initial referral and subsequent treatment can greatly influence the patient's outlook or attitude. Remember, pain generally produces a fear response. If the fear response is recognized early and treated appropriately it can assist in mitigating subsequent emotional consequences.

I suspect that most difficult or unmotivated patients are the conditioned result of repetitive negative treatment outcomes. The hope or optimism that may exist in the beginning stages is negatively conditioned over time and results in despair and pessimism. Pain medicine by its nature is a trial and error process. Therefore, the more negative trials the patient experiences, the more difficult and unmotivated they become. If providers recognize and understand this process early and incorporate the services of adjunctive support personnel, including the utilization of a pain psychologist, the outcomes can improve greatly.

The Referral Process

The primary care physician (PCP) usually has a number of options of where to refer the patient for more specialized pain care. These options can include private pain clinics, medical school based pain programs and the individual pain specialist. The referral may be further influenced by insurance coverage or location. In the rural setting, options may be limited unless the patient is willing to travel long distances.

The secondary referral to a pain specialist is an important step in the process whether it be for a diagnosis with a recommendation back to the primary care physician for follow-up care, or it could involve repeated visits for further invasive diagnostic procedures. It is important that at this point in the process the patient is introduced to adjunctive support care.

When I was part of a medical school pain program the patient was required to be evaluated by all of the adjunctive staff including a board certified pain physician, psychologist and physical therapist. The advantage of the multidisciplinary pain program is that all issues impacting the patient are addressed early and are incorporated into a comprehensive treatment program. If the patient has a positive and supportive experience, then the potential for hope is reinforced and counterproductive issues such as anger and frustration are mitigated. If the secondary referral is based on the premise that I have nothing further to offer, go see a pain specialist, the patient then feels like a failure and the trial and error process of negative reinforcement begins.

Over the past 30 years I have experienced many types of referrals. If my services are incorporated early in the treatment process, then I am more optimistic about the outcome. Unfortunately, this is not always the case, especially over the last 10 years as an independent provider operating in a hostile insurance environment. Many of my referrals have been in the trial and error treatment process with repetitive failures. They often do not understand why they have to see a pain psychologist. Further, they feel that nobody believes their pain is "real" and by being referred to a pain psychologist that their pain is "all in their head" or imaginary. So by the time I saw the patient, he/she had already been characterized as being difficult and unmotivated.

The Initial Visit

The initial visit is critical in establishing a connection with the patient. When I was the psychologist at the pain management clinic at OHSU, patients went through a full day of psychometric testing. Over the nine years I was at the pain center, I accumulated over 2000 profiles. The data from these patients were presented at numerous national and international pain meetings throughout the 90s. Subsequently, as a solo practitioner, I did not have the luxury of administering a large psychometric battery. For the past 10 years I have relied on the clinical interview as my main source of data. Early in my career, I experience a wonderful week-long workshop with Wilbur Fordyce, PhD. He shared his Behavioral Analysis of Pain (BAP), which I still incorporate into my initial interview. (See Chapter 3 on for more information on the BAP.) One additional comment I would like to mention is that I avoid offering a psychological pain diagnosis in my report to the referring physician. Most psychological pain diagnoses are not well understood and are not based on current accepted empirical standards. Instead I offer my clinical impression where I attempt to point out the issues that may be influencing the patient's pain, including both strengths and weaknesses.

In addition, I use Melzack's model of chronic pain during my initial evaluation in identifying both affective and cognitive factors that are influencing the patient's perception of pain. For a more detailed discussion of Melzack's model, I would refer the reader to my article published in the March 2013 issue of *Practical Pain Management* (*PPM*). Keep in mind that a considerable number of pain patients are clinically depressed by the time they are initially evaluated by a pain specialist.

I have seen ranges from a low of 60% to a high of 80%. Depression results from profound feelings of learned hopelessness and helplessness. As the patient experiences repetitive treatment failures, this sense of despair accumulates which, in my opinion, forms the basis of why the patient appears unmotivated.

So how do I, as a pain psychologist, start to treat a depressed, unmotivated patient? The first step is my assessment of the patient's strengths and weaknesses. Are they open and at least curious about the nature of their pain? Are they willing to accept that they are responsible for practicing the recommended treatments on their own outside their doctors' offices?

From a cognitive behavioral treatment perspective, this is a crucial first step, and I have learned over the years that this may not be accomplished in the first session. The patient needs to trust me and realize that I am not going to question the validity of their pain. Many patients are cautious and somewhat dubious, especially after experiencing repeated treatment failures.

I believe there are many levels of trust and I will continue to build trust as treatment progresses. One technique that I have used throughout my career to build trust is that I will call the patient at home to check on how they are doing. I also give the patient my personal cell number and encourage them to call me if they have a concern or question. I have never experienced a patient abusing this privilege and it facilitates trust building. I am very careful about building trust and not dependence, which I consider counterproductive to the desired treatment process.

Information Sharing

The next phase of treatment is what I call information sharing. Knowledge is a powerful tool that will help the patient begin to achieve some sense of self-control. I often use the metaphor of the pain management tool box and share with the patient that all of their providers have tools to add to the tool box. The more tools the patient has the better able they are able to control their pain and subsequently improve the quality of their life.

One of the tools that I use is an excellent workbook titled *Managing Your Pain Before it Manages You*, by Margaret Caudill, MD, PhD, MPH.[2] It discusses the nature of pain, procedures and treatment procedures in language that most patients understand and appreciate. In addition, I also see it as a test of motivation. Will they read it and more importantly will they do the exercises suggested in this workbook?

Because of my interest in applied psychophysiology and biofeedback, I spend a considerable amount of time discussing the sympathetic nervous system and its relationship to pain. There is a large body of research supporting the fact that if you lower your sympathetic reactivity you will lower your pain level. In other words, if I can teach the patient to self-control the sympathetic response by utilizing relaxation techniques augmented by biofeedback, they now possess a powerful tool to control their pain. The more perceived self-control the patient has over their pain the more their feelings of helplessness and hopelessness will subside. Early in my career I utilized many biofeedback modalities including respiration, EMG, EDR and skin temperature. All of these modalities were recorded and charted by the use of a computer. In addition, I used computer games tied into sympathetic self-control.

Today I have simplified this treatment modality and now focus on one indicator of sympathetic reactivity. Peripheral skin temperature feedback is reliable and easy for the patient to understand. More importantly, they can use it at home and work by the use of skin thermometer, which costs about $1.50. If I can teach the patient to raise their skin temperature by just a few degrees and trigger the relaxation response, the patient will usually report a lower pain level. I also recommend Herbert Benson's classic book, *The Relaxation Response,* to my patients.[1] It provides excellent understandable knowledge about how our physiology works and how we can control our sympathetic arousal.

Relaxation Therapy

I would like to share some thoughts that have been formed by using relaxation therapy augmented by biofeedback over the past 30 years. My approach emphasizes relaxation therapy as the primary modality, which is augmented or reinforced by adding biofeedback. The treatment algorithm I employ starts with teaching the patient to diaphragmatically breathe. Most pain patients use shallow breaths and will hold their breath when they experience a pain episode. This action coupled with physical tensing and bracing will increase their pain level. If I can teach the patient to breathe diaphragmatically through this pain episode, they will achieve a beginning sense of self-control over their pain. If they can slow their respiration rate to under 12 breaths per/minute, they are now able to begin the process of achieving the relaxation response. A general word of caution regarding diaphragmatic breathing techniques: as the CO_2 level changes, the patient may feel dizzy or lightheaded, therefore, they should be well supported in a chair or a bed, and never use these techniques when driving or operating heavy machinery.

The next step in my treatment algorithm is to introduce the patient to progressive relaxation. This technique has been around a long time and it is easy to learn. It is based on isometric contraction, tensing muscle groups, then releasing the tension. After repetitive trials the muscles will relax. In addition, I will pair deep diaphragmatic breathing with the tensing/relaxing exercise. As the patient tenses the muscle the patient inhales a slow deep breath through the nose, expanding the chest, holding the breath for a few seconds, then exhaling through the mouth, releasing and blowing away the tension. I will also use the visualization of blowing up a balloon with their pain and then letting it float up into the sky letting it disappear. The visualization of blowing up the balloon helps the patient empty their lungs. A word of caution when using progressive relaxation with pain patients: if it hurts to tense any muscle group, then I ask the patient to avoid that muscle group. I will address painful muscle groups later in the treatment sequence when I introduce visualization and autogenic techniques.[3]

If the patient does well with diaphragmatic breathing and progressive relaxation and they appear open to more abstract techniques, I will then introduce autogenic therapy. This is also a well-known and successful technique that is based on self-phasing using themes of "heavy and warm". I also consider autogenics as a preliminary step to self-hypnosis. It is more effective if the patient takes some time preparing their body by using diaphragmatic breathing and progressive relaxation to lower their level of arousal. The more relaxed the patient is the more likely the self-phasing will have the desired impact. The brain will be more open to the self-suggestions. If the patient completes the autogenic phase and wishes to experience a deeper level of relaxation, I will add a simple induction procedure. Now the patient has progressed to self-hypnosis that they can use by themselves in their world without my presence. The next logical step is having the patient join a meditation support group, which will help to promote maintenance.

As I mentioned earlier, relaxation skills are powerful tools that the patient can use the rest of their lives to help control pain, promote sleep and improve immune response. The main premise of these therapeutic approaches is to give the patient a perceived sense of control over their pain. This sense of control helps to counter feelings of hopelessness and helplessness. Further, feelings of hopelessness and helplessness are what I see as the main ingredients in the profile of the unmotivated patient.

Summary

I have provided a snapshot of the pain psychologist's role in the multidisciplinary approach to chronic pain. The unmotivated patient presents a difficult and unique challenge that takes time and patience to change. The pain psychologist can provide valuable insight and assistance in working with the unmotivated patient. Hopefully, I have stimulated primary care and pain physicians to realize that the referral process is critical in shaping the patient's attitude toward treatment. Repeated treatment failures have a profound effect, which in many cases could be avoided. How treatment failures are addressed is a critical step and with the use of adjunctive support early in the treatment process as pain specialists will achieve more treatment successes.

Chapter

10 Pain and Physical Therapy

THIS CHAPTER INCLUDES A STORY ABOUT MY OWN EXPERIENCE with acute pain, followed by an in-depth interview with Brad Simpson, Doctor of Physical Therapy. Dr. Simpson also discusses posture and body awareness.

The Role of Physical Therapy in Pain Management

A Personal Experience

Last winter I experienced an acute back injury that resulted in severe low back pain. It was difficult to stand or walk without pain. At first, I thought the cause was back strain or muscle spasm. But since I was also experiencing radiating pain into my right hip, I was suspicious.

I was scheduled to leave for Southern California for a month of sun and golf. So I thought a little rest in a long car trip would help. With the help of ibuprofen and stretching, I made it from Portland to Palm Springs. It was not getting better.

I then went in to the Eisenhower Immediate Care Center where I met a wonderful physician by the name of Denny Mauricio, MD. After his careful assessment, he prescribed Tramadol, 50 mg, three times a day, and Carisoprodol at bedtime to help with sleep. In addition, he administered a shot of Toradal IM and a referral to the Eisenhower Medical Center for a lumbar MRI. I scheduled a follow up for the next week where I learned the results of my MRI. The results were remarkable for degenerative lumbar disc disease plus three bulging discs at L3/4, 4/5 and 5/S1. The L4/5 disc bulge was the most significant which explained the radiating pain into my right hip.

It was an awkward situation since my visit was limited, but Dr. Mauricio agreed to see me weekly for my Toradal injections. Over the next three weeks, I tried to practice what I preach; which involved relaxation exercises and stretches in the hot tub, but no golf. Toward the end of three weeks my pain started to subside so I headed home to rain and cold weather, which did not help.

When I got home I scheduled a visit with Ruhul Desi, MD, an interventional radiologist who runs a clinic called Restore PDX. I wanted him to look at my MRI and give me an opinion. He recommended physical therapy and referred me to an excellent physical therapist by the name of Brad Simpson. I should mention that I have always been a strong supporter of physical therapy going back to my time at OHSU where we had a dedicated physical therapist in our pain management program who evaluated every referral. I knew right away that Brad was very knowledgeable, so I asked him if he would be willing to co-write an article on the role of physical therapy in the management of pain. He agreed, and we decided on the format of a series of questions and answers regarding the current role of physical therapy in the management of pain. Some of the questions are fairly specific and some are general, which gave him more latitude in formulating his answers.

I worked with Brad for 12 weeks at 2 times per week. At the end of 12 weeks of therapy, my back pain had subsided from the severe range of 8/10 to the mild range of 2/10 and I started playing golf and tennis again. I still do my stretches and I am limiting my swing in both golf and tennis, but it feels good to be back in the game!

Over the course of my rehabilitation, I considered a surgical consultation, but my common sense said to hold off and trust my body to repair itself with the help of physical therapy.

Q & A with Dr. Olson and Dr. Brad Simpson

Kern A. Olson, PhD Clinical Health Psychologist Pain Management, posed a series of questions to Brad Simpson, DPT, CSCS, COMT, FAAOMPT. The following discussion is the result.

1. What made you want to become a physical therapist? People who influenced you, why you chose your training program?

I knew in high-school that I wanted to get in a profession where I could help people. I shadowed various healthcare professions, and felt physical therapy was the best fit for me. It seemed to be a well-respected healthcare profession, and I was told how it was in a growing need due to an aging population and healthcare changes. Physical therapy is truly a positive profession, in that we have the benefit of seeing people 'get better' every day. For the small population I feel I am not helping get better, I can help those people get to other healthcare professionals with the hopes of getting them on the right path towards improvement. Our mission is to help maximize people's potential, which is an amazing goal to strive for every day.

2. Talk about your background, experience and education, and how this has changed in the past few years.

I graduated from Oregon State University in 2002, with a B.S. in Exercise & Sports Science. I graduated from Pacific University in 2005 with a Doctorate of Physical Therapy.

From the start of my career, I have been fortunate to have brilliant mentors who taught me to continue learning, and to always ask the question 'why' with patients. For example, after examining a person with insidious onset left-sided knee pain, I would be challenged by mentors with questions such as, 'why did this happen to his left side, not his right side?' I was educated early on of the benefits of residency or fellowship, and got introduced to the North American Institute of Orthopedic Manual Physical Therapy (NAIOMT), which is where I completed my manual therapy Fellowship in 2012.

Throughout my career, it has been interesting seeing how some people improve and others have a more difficult time, when rehabbing from what seems to be the same condition. For the majority of my career, I worked in a clinic that attracted a high percentage of complex, chronic pain patients, and I began adopting a more Biopsychosocial model for treating clients. When a person becomes injured, the Fear-Avoidance Model (FAM) suggests there are two paths a patient's recovery process can take, depending on psychological factors such as negative affect, threatening illness information, pain catastrophizing, fear of pain, and pain anxiety. If these variables are not present, normal recovery takes place. If they are present, there is a higher likelihood of fear-avoidance behaviors which may lead towards chronic musculoskeletal pain syndromes. So, even though there are biological issues still needing addressing, there are also psychosocial aspects that may be affecting the patient's ability to properly heal. Unless these barriers to successful rehabilitation are addressed, the patient will likely not improve, or struggle with long-term success.

Another main concept emphasized through my fellowship was foundation-building. It was stressed to me that "good physical therapists do the simple things well." In addressing patients with chronic pain, this concept helped when I realized these patients were simply not 'managing well'. They have no foundation to progress from, and continue to hit a wall every time they try to progress. I began helping them form foundations, normalizing their 'normal' prior to progressing their home program. Our body is so good at compensating when it is in pain; it is part of our survival. If those compensation patterns are not addressed and improved, it does not matter what we do with that patient, their pain is likely going to come back. So, with every patient, both acute and chronic, I look to first normalize patterns, get them functioning their normal life more normal, prior to implementing a larger-scale home program. Then, we have something to build on. If we hit a wall later in rehab, we have something to fall back on. The patient's fear stays low knowing they have an independent way to manage their pain to get back towards their baseline, which is empowering.

3. Explain all those letters behind your name.

I am a Doctor of Physical Therapy, or DPT. Every physical therapy-accredited school in the U.S. is now a DPT program, which was the Vision 2020 goal of the American Physical Therapy Association (APTA) in 2000. This DPT became a focus as the APTA was legislating for patients to be able to see physical therapists through Direct Access, or without the need of a physician referral. Now, every state in the U.S. has at least some form of direct access.

I successfully completed all the requirements of the NAIOMT clinical fellowship program in 2012, and received my COMT, which is a Certified Orthopaedic Manipulative Therapist. I also received the designation of Fellow (FAAOMPT) through the American Academy of Orthopaedic Manual Physical Therapists (AAOMPT) in 2012. I am also a CSCS, which is a Certified Strength and Conditioning Specialist.

4. Talk about your initial evaluation, what do you look for? And do you approach chronic and acute pain differently?

During my initial evaluation, the first thing I do is look at the patient chart, giving me an idea of gender, age, location of pain, duration of symptoms, and any other information available, such as Fear-Avoidance Belief Questionnaire score (FABQ). Even before greeting the patient I begin building hypotheses that I will look to confirm or negate with the examination. On the first day, I spend a good portion of the evaluation talking to the client and hearing what they think is going on. If I get a sense the patient has apprehension for physical therapy, or high fear along with their chronic pain, I may not perform much objective assessment on day one. If this patient appears to be appropriate for therapy, I may go right into pain education and how I plan to address their case. I would discuss how we will do more assessing in future visits, and continue to look at things depending on how they respond to the treatment. The last thing I want to do is put a chronic pain patient in more pain until they have bought-in, and trust, me as someone who is going to help them improve. This is different than someone who has low fear and acute symptoms. I can go right into the objective examination with these patients, and possibly treat them with more manual therapy or physical treatment without going into much detail on pain education.

5. As you look back, what is the most prevalent pain condition that is referred for physical therapy?

Low back pain is a societal epidemic, and is poorly managed, evidenced by the extreme amount of money spent treating it in the U.S. annually. Most low back pain is chronic, comes and goes, and 50% of people in our society have it on an annual basis. I feel it is a difficult region to treat with long-term success, without taking a biopsychosocial approach to its management. The likelihood is that even if the person's painful episode goes away (which it likely will), there is a large chance that the pain will come back at some point in the future. People with low back pain need to be educated on their back, how to improve themselves to minimize future episodes, and how to self-manage their pain in the future. Though future low back pain is likely eminent, how the person responds to it, how often it recurs, how quickly it resolves, and the ability to continue improving over the long term can all be effected by how a painful episode is conservatively managed.

6. What are yellow flags to you that a patient who has acute symptoms may be at risk of becoming a chronic pain patient?

I look at the Fear-Avoidance Belief Questionnaire (FABQ) and see where they lie on the scale that tells me how they perceive their pain, how fearful they are about resuming their activities, and what their perceptions are about their likelihood of getting better. Fear has been shown to be the number one predictor of chronic pain. The FABQ has been shown to be a reliable tool identifying individuals who are likely going to take longer to improve, or who will have a hard time getting back to their normal activities because of fear and anxiety of their pain. It can be used with patients who have chronic symptoms, where if they score high on the FABQ I make sure we focus some of the education on chronic pain to help decrease their fear and anxiety. If the patient's condition is acute, and they score high on the FABQ, that fear/anxiety may contribute to that person becoming a chronic pain patient, so I make sure we address chronic pain with this person also.

I pay attention to various yellow flag responses during the interview process. Chronic pain patients may state how everything hurts and no position provides comfort. Or, they state they have had multiple practitioners treat the same condition, with numerous tests completed, tried various medications, and/or tried other procedures, all without helping. The more the patient has had done, the more passive procedures that have not changed their course of treatment, the more concerned I am. When nothing helps, it tells me they have poor self-management of their symptoms. Also, if the patient seems like their painful part is a person, with a name for it or references it like a he or she, those are not normal responses.

Some other yellow flags during the interview can be their past history of pain, how it was treated, how long it took to get better and what they did to improve, and their feelings towards those previous injuries. These answers may give insight to their current condition, and how their body likely will respond to the pain.

7. Do you address ergonomics with chronic pain patients?

I address ergonomics with anyone who performs the same thing over and over in their job, or who stays in one position for long-durations, which seems to be most people. Frequently, I hear patients state their pain gets worse during work, or as the week goes on, and is better during the weekends and vacations. Those statements are clues that ergonomics needs to be addressed.

Simply put, ergonomics is the art of finding the ideal position for your body and building your environment around that ideal. Too often, people are forced to mold themselves to an environment that is not ideal for them and, over time, their body begins to hurt because of it.

I always ask patients during the interview what makes their pain feel better or worse. Musculoskeletal pain has a mechanical nature to it – certain activities affect it differently. I have noticed a trend with chronic pain patients. They commonly state various activities do feel better with work, such as pulling their shoulder blades back, stretching their arms up and overhead, or getting up and walking around, to name a few. When asked what prompted them to do that 'feel good' activity, they would tell me it was due to pain. This is where I feel people can fall into problems. If your body waits for 'pain', you have waited too long to make your correction. Normal (people without chronic pain) people frequently shift and stretch throughout the day also. The difference, however, is that normal people don't typically realize they are doing it, and their body is not with pain when they do it. Their bodies are aware of position, and too much time in one position gets their bodies to subconsciously move. Chronic pain patients focus on the pain, and react to it by moving instead of being proactive and learning how to respond to position instead of waiting until pain worsens. This is the hard part, as this proactive approach towards change takes thousands of repetitions and a lot of mental focus. It is changing a mindset from one focusing on pain to one recognizing position. Chronic pain is literally a state where you are always in a 'fight or fight'. They need to learn how to get out of the fight and begin letting their bodies relax.

Years ago, I designed an example of a bell curve that I show to chronic pain patients, describing where I hope they get to over time. Rather than being a patient depicted on the bottom of the curve, focusing on 'pain' and reacting to pain with extreme measures before going right back to the positions that bother him/her, I want their body to be sensitive to 'position', which is at the example at the top of the bell curve. Feel good postures are great to have in your belt, and using them when you need to is healthy. It is not healthy, however, if it is a constant response to pain. If pain starts after 30 minutes of sitting, I want that person moving at 15 minutes. That is a positive response to position, and telling the body that doing this feels good, recognizing that the previous position would likely not be comfortable if stayed in for long duration.

It takes literally thousands of repetitions to change a body's habits to shift from pain to position-sense, but it begins to empower patients to be proactive instead of reactive. Think of the people you see fidgeting all the time. When I see this, it is likely due to something hurting. Fidgeting is an attempt to get comfortable. But, it is not solving anything. What do people do after they fidget? They go right back to the same position that caused them to feel like they needed to fidget again. The next time they want to fidget, I tell them to correct their posture, to relax, and comfortably breathe. When they want to fidget again, I tell them to correct the posture again and work on relaxed breathing. Throughout the day, I am fine with stretching, frequent breaks, and building an environment suitable for each person's own needs. A frequent goal for patients is to come back saying they feel they do not need to fidget as often anymore.

8. What are you looking for to show signs of early progress with chronic pain patients?

I look for a patient's wording in how they describe their painful condition to change first. Not to sound cliché, but I want a patient telling me what they can do instead of just focusing on what they cannot do. When you have chronic pain, you focus on pain, and it may be difficult to sense progress.

For example, a patient initially states their pain is 8/10, on a scale of 0–10, with 10/10 pain being the worst pain imaginable. This person may state at future visits that their pain is still 8/10, if you only ask them what their pain level is. So, does this mean the person is not improving? Possibly, this person may have a pain that indeed spikes to 8/10, but they are able to get the pain down by doing "x" now. If the pain was present 50% of their day, for example, now it may be present only 30% of the day, which is an improvement. Because of this, I ask more questions about function and their exercises, and see how the patient responds.

9. How do you address the pain word with chronic pain patients?

I rarely use the word 'pain' with chronic pain patients. Early on, I may use it as I educate them about chronic pain and the processes that are occurring which I feel may be affecting their ability to properly heal. I ask patients "How're your exercises?" instead of "How's your pain?" Other examples are, "How have things been since our last visit?" or "How is traction appearing to help?" At the onset of treatment, many patients are not aware that certain things help them feel better; they just think everything hurts. So, starting to have them focus on things that feel better helps them realize there is hope, and begins getting them to focus on something other than pain. As treatment progresses, I look for these patients to use the word pain less often.

10. How do you communicate with other providers who are treating these patients with chronic pain?

I try to keep open communication lines with my referring providers, mostly regarding chronic pain patients. These patients have frequent follow-ups with the other providers, and it is important we are all using the same language, have the same goals, and are being told the same things from the patient. I want to understand the physician's medication plans for both short-term and long-term, and how those are being monitored. Chronic pain patients frequently come in on multiple medications to help manage their pain, which the physician is addressing. My input on how PT is being tolerated may help determine how the physician tapers the patient off of certain medications.

Dr. Brad Simpson on Posture and Body Awareness

Individuals with chronic pain shift frequently from poor postures to extreme-opposite postures throughout the day, waiting until the pain increases to make a change, then quickly returning to the extreme poor position after the feel-good activity subsides.

This strategy bypasses any ideal position that allows their body to relax, and fails to provide the person with positive learning, since it is always reactive to their pain.

People without chronic pain also tend towards poor posture throughout the day. However, due to improved positional sense, they subconsciously move before pain occurs, and will either stretch, or improve their posture towards the 'ideal posture' range for a given time period, allowing their body to relax. This strategy is proactive, promoting positive learning by sensing position in order to promote change, instead of only responding to pain.

Body awareness determines behavior. It is not about being 'perfect' but rather about training your body to be aware of position and correct posture due to position-sense, not pain. Having a work/life environment that allows you to be posturally 'ideal' is important.

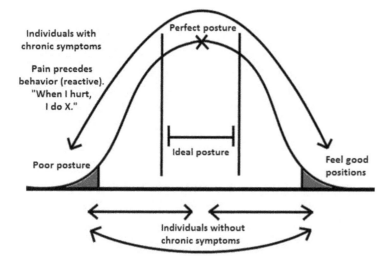

This posture curve, originated by Dr. Brad Simpson, depicts commonly-noted postural patterns and strategies from people who have chronic pain, versus people without chronic pain.

Conclusion

Pain can be scary. It triggers superstitious thinking that leads to fear. But knowledge is a powerful tool that helps to counteract the fear and discouragement that individuals often experience when they live with chronic or recurrent pain.

I believe pain patients have a natural drive to try to understand how their bodies work and why they experience chronic pain. We should never underestimate the patient's desire for knowledge or dismiss their level of curiosity in understanding the pain experience.

My hope is that this book will help the individual sufferer become his or her own best friend and advocate, and that health care providers who work with pain patients will gain insight into the practice of pain management and the vast complexity of pain experiences.

Case Studies

Case Studies and A Little Common Sense

THIS CHAPTER FOCUSES ON PATIENTS I HAVE EVALUATED AND TREATED over the past 20 years. The primary selection factor for inclusion is the uniqueness of the presenting pain. I considered whether or not the case presented a 'teachable moment' that would benefit the reader and I selected only cases that I treated for an extended period of time. Those cases that were simply evaluated or seen for a brief time were not included as they generally did not present enough information to demonstrate treatment efficacy.

The term "a little common sense" in the title of this chapter reflects the growth or evolution of my therapeutic approach to treatment. Early in my career, I was more technique oriented and theoretically exclusive. Even today I still lean toward the behavioral approach but I have learned through experience to be more flexible and more pragmatic. The spectrum of pain patients is highly variable and therefore the provider must tailor the treatment approach to fit the needs and personality of the patient. For example, certain patients may not want to talk about their pain and may prefer a more nonverbal approach or technique. On the other end of the spectrum there are patients who have a need to describe every nuance of their pain experience. What I have learned through my experience is that I needed to achieve a balance between active listening and directive problem solving. My personal approach to therapy as a pain psychologist is primarily knowledge- or education-based. The more a patient knows about their pain, the more power they have in managing their pain. In the chapter on the nature of pain, I mentioned that it can be a fearful and foreign experience, which is an anxiety-producing and counterproductive influence. So to me, the early phase of therapy is information-based which helps to build trust. If the patient does not learn to trust you, the therapy experience is likely to be short and a waste of time. Therapy is a process that requires both individuals, the patient and the provider, to fully engage in the give-and-take of the learning experience.

The more experience the provider has, the more they will trust their common sense. Every pain patient has a story to share and I have found over the years of practice that it is important for the patient to tell their story to an objective, compassionate audience. That story helps them validate what they are going through and that they are still worthwhile individuals.

I have also learned which patients to offer therapy services and which patients to refer to another provider. When I was at the pain center at OHSU, which is a publicly-funded medical school, we evaluated everyone who came through the door. Treatment options were offered, and voluntary, which in practical terms translated to some patients just wanting pain medication. Since we were a multidisciplinary pain center we had some leverage, so it was never just a pill. The pill was contingent on other treatment options, such as PT, OT, behavioral treatment, etc. In other words, the patient was expected to become a full participant in the treatment experience.

While at OHSU, I evaluated every referral to the pain center, plus, for two years, every patient referred to the neurosurgery pain center for consideration of implantable pain technology. Between the two pain programs, I estimate that I evaluated over 5,000 pain patients, some of whom would have also required extensive multidisciplinary pain treatment.

The following format will include a brief historical overview, including both medical and behavioral treatments. Rarely did I get the opportunity to participate early in the treatment process. This was a disappointing observation I learned both in the medical and private practice settings.

Typically, by the time I became involved, the pain patient had experienced multiple interventions and treatments. I estimated at one point in my career that 50% of my patients were failed back-surgery patients. The most extreme example was a gentleman who was referred by the state's workers' compensation program to evaluate and recommend if he was an appropriate candidate for another back surgery. He had undergone 12 previous back surgeries, all failed, and his neurosurgeon had convinced him that number 13 would "cure" him of his pain! I mention this caveat to the reader because most pain programs and pain specialists treat a heavily skewed sample of the total population of chronic pain patients. Not all pain treatments fail. If the patient has undergone a treatment or surgery that is successful there is no reason to refer them to a pain program or a pain specialist. Very little is known about the successful pain patient treatment outcome. It is an area that needs more research attention, because I believe we can learn from those patients.

I will describe in some depth the various treatments that each of the patients experienced from his or her point of view. To protect the privacy of the patients, no names will be used. Each case will be referred to by a number, and background information will be omitted if it could potentially reveal the identity of the patient being discussed.

Patient #1

This patient was pleasant to work with, highly motivated, and bright. He experienced a significant work injury and underwent a number of medical procedures, including multiple surgeries. He experienced extreme psychosocial distress for most of the time that I treated him.

When the patient was referred to me, he was in his early 40s. He described his early childhood as active and healthy, but mentioned that his father abused him physically and that his father was an alcoholic. He did well in school, graduating from high school in 1975. He admitted that he experiment with drugs and abused alcohol during his early teen years. He enlisted in the army and received an honorable discharge. After the army, he attended school and studied electronics. He accepted a position with a large telecommunication company, first as an installer, then worked his way up to supervisor over a period of 2 years.

When I initially evaluated him, he was going through a painful divorce. He had been married for 4 years. His wife had 3 children by a previous marriage and he described a close emotional relationship with his stepchildren. His wife was contesting any custody by the patient. Further, one of the daughters had terminal brain cancer and his ex-wife refused him visiting rights. To complicate matters more, his mother was also very ill with lung cancer.

His work injury resulted from a fall of approximately 30 feet from a telephone pole. He landed on his head and shoulder, resulting in multiple fractures of his cervical spine. He underwent surgery resulting in a cervical fusion that included hardware. He was treated medically for about a year, with significant pain persisting in his neck, and with pain and weakness radiating down his right arm into his hand. He underwent a second surgery with no pain relief. He described his pain as sharp and shooting and also reported constant headache.

I saw him about one year after his initial work injury and at that time his pain levels ranged from 7/10 to 10/10. He stated his pain was fairly constant but worse with activity.

Further, he described a serious sleep issue, stating he could sleep only 2 to 3 hours at a time due to pain. He related that he experienced daytime fatigue due to a lack of restorative sleep. At the time of my initial evaluation, he had been prescribed 60 mg of Oxycontin, plus Neurontin and Zanaflex. He said the medicine was helpful. He was also being considered for a trial of spinal cord stimulation.

My initial clinical impression was that he had a significant mood disorder, but I did not feel he was self-destructive. He also had a significant sleep disorder (insomnia) that was also compounding his mood disorder. Further, the psychosocial distress he was experiencing was contributing to his overall level of distress.

He was referred by a pain specialist, who had tried a number of injections including epidural steroids and an occipital nerve block with no lasting relief. He was also being treated by his primary care physician, who had known the patient for a very long time. I had a good working relationship with both physicians. He was not drug seeking and there were no outstanding personality issues. (AXIS II).

He was open to adjunctive behavioral treatment. He indicated that he was motivated and would be willing to be actively involved, which is supportive of a successful outcome. I usually request a homework assignment at the end of the first visit, mainly as a test of commitment to behavioral therapy.

The first assignment was to purchase a copy of *Managing Pain Before it Manages You*, by Margaret Caudill, MD, PhD. It is an excellent workbook and one that I first introduced when I was at the medical school. It is now in its fourth edition. The second assignment was a sleep log that basically involved self-monitoring a number of behaviors on a daily basis. The simple act of self-monitoring is a therapeutic technique, and it also provides useful information that can be incorporated into the treatment plan.

Before the second visit I contacted both of his treating physicians recommending that an anti-depressant medication be prescribed. His primary care physician was open to this suggestion and ordered 100mg of Elavil to be taken at bedtime.

At the beginning of treatment, I try to see the patient on a weekly basis depending on insurance limitations. I will admit that his workers' compensation insurance company was difficult to work with. They did not want to authorize adjunctive behavioral treatment since they felt his depression and sleep problems were not related to his injury. Therefore, it required all three providers writing multiple letters, as well as his attorney, before they agreed to authorize behavioral treatment. This process added further stress for the patient. In my opinion, stressors are additive and directly impact the patient's perceived level of pain and psychosocial distress.

In the second and subsequent sessions, I devoted at least 20 minutes to talking and active listening. He continued to be angry with his ex-wife for not allowing him to visit his stepdaughter in the hospital. She was not expected to live much longer, so it was important for him to vent his frustration, and I assumed an emotionally supportive position. I knew if we did not deal with his anger, other pain management techniques would fail. As he calmed down, I introduced some basic information about pain and what he could do by himself on his own time.

During the remainder of the sessions we talked about general relaxation approaches, including deep breathing, self-phasing, and visualization. He was open to relaxation techniques of tensing and relaxing various muscle groups with the caution he should avoid tensing his head and neck muscles since I did not want him to experience a muscle spasm. I also introduced temperature biofeedback at this point since he was cold in his extremities. The stress and anger he was experiencing fired up his sympathetic reactivity resulting in vasoconstricting. With his engineering background, he was fascinated by the numbers. I used a simple skin thermometer to measure his skin temperature and he was indicating temperatures in the low 80s. The benefit of the skin thermistor was he could take it with him and practice in his home environment or as he went about his day. It also helped reinforce the mind/body relationship and how an increase in skin temperature can lower pain levels.

After a couple of sessions, the patient reported he was still not sleeping well, so I called his primary care physician to share this feedback. His physician then DC'ed the Elavil and switched him to a starter pack of Effexor XR. After a couple of weeks he reported that his mood and sleep were improving. He was also practicing his relaxation techniques on a daily basis. His pain level still remained high at 7/10. I used the self-reported pain level as a projective measurement of his overall level of psychosocial distress. Also, at this time he was going to court over custody of his stepchildren and his right to visit his stepdaughter in the hospital. Consequently, his stress level was high which directly impacted his mood and pain levels. At this point, I introduced autogenic relaxation therapy, which involves self-phasing to enhance the overall effect. I have found from experience that not all patients respond well to autogenic therapy. Since this patient was bright and curious and could process more abstract techniques he responded well. If used properly with the appropriate patient, autogenics can be a powerful therapeutic tool and it opens the door to self-hypnosis.

I should also mention that I encouraged him to use heat while he was at home practicing his relaxation techniques, and stretching, which was introduced to him by his physical therapist. A simple and inexpensive way to achieve this is to fill an old tube sock with rice, tie it off with a rubber band and place it in the microwave for 2 minutes.

In June his stepdaughter passed away, which was a difficult period, especially since he had never received permission to visit her. So we spent the next session focused on grief, which was important for the patient since this was a major source of stress. It is important for the provider to recognize that psychosocial stressors play an important role in the therapeutic process, and at times it needed to be addressed, along with the primary pain management focus. I felt this detour was important for the patient and he appreciated the emotional support, which helped build more trust.

During this period the patient received permission from his workers' compensation insurance to proceed with a trial of spinal cord stimulation. His pain management physician felt it was important for him to at least go through the trial. Even though he had responded well to adjunctive behavioral therapy, his level of psychosocial stress remained high. I expressed serious reservations. Needless to say, the trial did not go well. He achieved at most a 20% reduction in his pain. His pain management physician then proposed a spinal trial of opioids. A spinal trial of opioids is a fairly straight-forward procedure and if the patient responds favorably it usually leads to the implantation of an intrathecal pump. The spinal trial did not go well. A miscommunication with the nurse administering the spinal trial resulted in an overdose of spinal opioids and the patient spent the next 3 days in critical care until he was stabilized. Unfortunately, this resulted in more anger and the patient wanted to sue the pain physician for malpractice. Since the patient now trusted me, I convinced him that more litigation would be counterproductive and would only increase his level of psychosocial distress and pain. I did help him find another pain physician and he agreed to write a personal letter to his pain physician explaining why he was transferring his pain care to a new physician and would he please forward his medical records.

His new pain physician discontinued his Oxycontin and started him on a trial of Methadone. He responded well to Methadone, which was titrated up to 75mg/daily with no central nervous system side effects. By this time, he was coming in about every two weeks, and his pain levels improved to 6/10. He reported improved sleep and his affect was brighter. He continued practicing his relaxation and stretching in his new hot tub. His new pain physician thought he would be a good candidate for Botox injections and he did receive some short-term relief. The focus of behavioral therapy consisted of emotional support and problem solving, based on cognitive behavioral techniques, mainly reframing negative thought patterns. I also encouraged him to be more socially and physically active.

After about a year of behavioral and medical therapy, his workers' compensation provider requested an independent medical examination (IME) to include a functional capacity evaluation. In the State of Oregon workers' compensation laws permit the use of an independent medical examination (IME) by a physician of the insurance company's choice. I have argued with various state officials, some elected and some appointed, that this is an unfair experience for the injured worker since these IME physicians are paid by the insurance carrier and therefore are not independent. It is an unfortunate law that requires the injured worker obtaining the services of an attorney. This adversarial process is highly stressful and results in the patient becoming the everlasting victim. All of his providers, including myself, wrote numerous letters, filled out repeated evaluations all stating that the patient was not medically stationary and that he was permanently disabled. As expected, his IME examination stated he could return to work and that his depression and sleep disorder were not related to his work injury. When I work with a patient who is injured either by work or an MVA, I will at times act as an advocate for the patient. I feel it as part of my ethical professional responsibility since the system is unfairly biased against the victim. All of his providers petitioned the state insurance commissioner who intervened on behalf of the patient and his disability payments were reinstated. All of his uncertainty about receiving his compensation pay added more stress and anxiety on top of the stressors I have previously mentioned. It was no wonder that his pain levels remained high and that his mood level was contributory to his overall level of psychosocial distress.

I continued to work with the patient over the next year on a fairly regular basis. We continued to work on the cognitive aspect of his pain and distress. We moved on to adding self-hypnosis by adding a simple induction procedure, which deepened his level of relaxation. I also used positive self-affirmations, explaining that in a relaxed state the brain is more open to absorb the positive self-statements. He was responding well to behavioral treatment and many of the stressors had subsided. He was reacting to or appraising stress in a more adaptive manner. Therapy during this time focused more on maintenance and shifted to a monthly schedule. He also met a new woman during this time that resulted in marriage. His new marriage seemed to stabilize the patient and approximately one year later they had a baby girl. They brought her in for my inspection, which as proud new parents they couldn't resist. She was absolutely precious and my patient was a natural at parenting. He became the primary caregiver since his new wife was attending school. His focus shifted from pain and disability to caring for his daughter. His mood improved and he became less dependent on his pain medicine.

The following year he informed me that he was moving to the east coast so his wife could attend school on a scholarship. He still calls me to give me updates and ask for advice. This was a pleasant outcome for me, since I was not optimistic about his prognosis at the beginning of our relationship. I was extremely gratified that he defied the odds.

Patient #2

I included this patient for discussion since I knew him well and he described a fairly complicated medical history. When I first evaluated him as a result of a referral from a local pain management physician, he was in his 40s. He was initially referred for pain management by a spine surgeon after numerous failed back surgeries.

His first spine surgeon performed an L4-5 partial discectomy with brief relief that lasted for only two months. He also received physical therapy during this period, with no relief. After an acute episode, he was referred to another spine surgeon who repeated the L4-5 discectomy without significant improvement. His pain persisted and he was referred to another spine surgeon who performed a foraminotomy at L4-5 with surgical scar revision. Also during this period, he was prescribed Oxycontin, Flexeril, and Neurontin with very little relief. He was then referred to a new spine surgeon who performed an L4-5 fusion and then 2 years later a new level fusion at L5-S1. During this period of multiple surgeries he continued to have low back pain with radiating leg pain.

During this period of multiple surgeries, his pain management physician performed numerous injections and trialed multimodal therapies. Included in these trials were two trials of spinal cord stimulators with little or no relief. He eventually went through a spinal trial of opioids (morphine) with 50% relief. He subsequently received an intrathecal pump and was managed on morphine for two years. He was then switched to Dilaundid which resulted in improved pain relief that also included oral opioids for breakthrough pain. His pain levels during this period while on the pump ranged from 3/10 to 9/10. He described his pain as stabbing in the low back with tingling and numbness down both legs. The only pain relief he experienced was lying supine. Aggravating factors included weight bearing (standing for prolonged periods) and truncal flexion.

During this time, I was also treating the patient with various behavioral therapies including relaxation therapy augmented by biofeedback and cognitive behavioral therapy. My clinical impression was significant mood swings that were directly related to pain relief. He was open to treatment both medical and psychological, as well as physical therapy in a warm therapeutic pool. He had worked for a large technology-based company and was receiving disability benefits. He was living with a woman and described a close supportive relationship. There were no children involved but a number of dogs. Psychosocial stressors were persistent pain, loss of a work identity, and a mother who was not well. He also had an older brother who was very successful financially and he described a close, emotionally supportive relationship with him as well.

He was trialed on numerous medications (oral) including Neurontin, Ambien, and Benedryl for sleep, and antidepressants, including Wellbutrin and Prozac. Both were discontinued due to cognitive issues. Additionally, he had experienced other surgeries including his left foot, left shoulder, and a right knee replacement. All of these medical procedures added more physical and emotional stress that compromised his quality of life. Financially, he was doing okay with disability, and his new wife worked as a long haul truck driver. He tried to remain active and optimistic about the future. He remained active in outpatient behavioral therapy and he felt it was helpful. Recently, he was trialed on Cymbalta, with positive results and continues at 60 mg/day. His intrathecal and oral opiates provided approximately sixty percent pain relief with mild, central side effects. His mood had stabilized.

Another important factor was that the patient described an ongoing sleep problem. As I mentioned in the chapter on Sleep and Pain, sleep issues are quite common with chronic pain patients, and because of this history, I referred the patient for a complete sleep study. His Epworth Sleepiness score was elevated to 14 and his wife rated him at 19. He also had a history of snoring and according to his wife he would stop breathing during the night. His polysomnography testing revealed sleep efficiency reduced to 80%, total sleep time of 181 minutes, sleep onset at 7 minutes with no REM (Rapid Eye Movement) sleep. Sleep staging was fragmented with 2% at Stage 1, 65% at Stage 2, 34% at Stage 3, and Stage 4 with no REM sleep, with increased alpha intrusions. His respiratory disturbance index was severely elevated. He exhibited obstructive hyponeas and apneas that were mixed and central with the longest at 41 seconds. He was diagnosed with central apnea syndrome and was prescribed a CPAP device. He responded well and his overall sleep improved with less daytime fatigue.

Based on my own experience and training in sleep, two issues are worth noting. First, the absence of REM sleep is clinically significant. It suggests he was experiencing no dream activity, which is important in maintaining emotional balance. Further, it is well known that some pain and sleep medications suppress REM sleep. The other issue is the increase in alpha intrusions, which suggest increased arousals that will compromise deep restorative sleep. There is also research support to suggest that increased alpha intrusions are associated with chronic pain, especially fibromyalgia. It also suggests increased sympathetic reactivity, which is consistent with vasoconstriction noted during my initial evaluation of this patient.

The patient exhibited a number of personality traits that contributed to his history of multiple failed surgeries. It is not the outcome of the multiple surgeries, but the fact that he received multiple failed surgeries. He is a pleasant and open fellow who was also highly compliant with treatment suggestions both medical and psychological.

It is important to consider whether all of these surgeries were necessary. Once a patient commits to seeking surgical relief, it is difficult to say no to subsequent surgical procedures, especially if pain relief is offered.

The costs of elective surgery in the US have risen dramatically over the past few years and now contribute to an overinflated financial burden that impacts every consumer of health care. Further, it relates to an earlier criticism that pain medicine is overly influenced by Cartesian Dualism, which has not been supported by empirical research.

My last contact with this patient was a phone call a couple of months ago. He shared that his quality of life had improved, he was more active, required less oral pain medicine, and that his pump was providing pain relief. He thanked me for advocating for him when times were bad. I should mention that when a patient terminates treatment, I always offer an open door policy; they can call me at any time.

I included this patient's case study because, in hindsight, he admitted that the rush to surgery was a mistake. He wished he had taken some time to let his body heal before he underwent the first surgery. The keynote here is to try conservative treatments first and let time take its course as the body heals itself.

Patient #3

This patient's case was interesting for many reasons. First, it was medically and psychologically complicated. Second, I saw this patient for over 10 years and therefore knew him well. At first he was reserved and suspicious. He did not like talking especially about himself. He was a stereotypic "down to earth kind of blue-collar guy" with black and white thinking, and therefore, was a challenge when it came to using adjunctive cognitive behavioral treatment. Generally, I am not a long-term therapy kind of psychologist, but this case showed me that long-term therapy had value for a select few patients. It was beneficial not only for emotional support, but also for ongoing problem-solving and maintenance.

At this time in my history, I was a solo practitioner, independently sharing office space with two rheumatologists. It was a very rewarding relationship as they were both very supportive of the multidisciplinary approach to treating pain, and I learned a lot from them. I found out that rheumatology basically treated very difficult and complex cases, especially fibromyalgia.

This case was a referral from one of my office partners. At the time of the referral, the patient was 55. He was born in Portland and grew up in Montana. His early health history was unremarkable until age 14, and there was no reported history of abuse. He attended public school and graduated from high school. He did not describe any problems in school, but described himself as a loner. He denied any history of drug or alcohol abuse.

At age 14 he accidentally shot himself in the head with a 22. He underwent surgery that repaired the damage, but the surgeon decided the safe course of action was to leave the bullet alone. The surgery resulted in a steel plate placed where the surgeon attempted to remove the bullet. He then experienced occasional seizure activity and headache. At age 14, he experienced chronic head pain that would last a lifetime.

After completing high school, he went to work with his father learning the trade of heavy construction. He worked with his father for three years at which time they discontinued his seizure control medicine and he has been seizure free, but with continued periodic headache. He then worked in the cleaning industry for 12 years before applying for and receiving social security disability income.

The patient has been married twice and his current wife, at the time of the initial evaluation was 53. They had three children, two daughters and a son, and he described a close relationship with his family. His wife works as a nurse at a care facility. I should also mention that he took care of a sister who had serious health issues, including fibromyalgia and chronic obstructive pulmonary disease (COPD). His sister was a constant source of stress, especially during the time she lived with him.

In his mid-twenties, he described the onset of depression and anger issues. He was treated with both inpatient and outpatient therapy, plus he was prescribed 40 mg of Paxil. He reported that both therapies were helpful in improving his mood and controlling his anger. At the time of the referral, he had been diagnosed with fibromyalgia, headache, depression, and low back pain. Plus, he was a pack a day smoker and experienced periodic asthma. At the time of his initial evaluation, he rated his pain at 5/10 with a range of 2/10 to 10/10. He reported that he experienced pain all over his body, but rated his back pain as number 1 with headache number 2. His pain management physician prescribed a Duragesic patch and Trazadone 50 mg at bedtime. At this time his rheumatologist had assumed the role of primary care provider and prescribed Tylenol #3, his heart meds, plus a muscle relaxer (Flexaril 10 mg x2 per day). He described his medicine as helpful but sleep issues persisted due to pain and breathing issues. Since his PCP and I shared an office suite, communication was enhanced by almost daily sharing of information about this patient. We both agreed that a full sleep study was indicated based on the patient's description of his poor sleep due to pain, possible breathing issues, and daytime fatigue, all of which were compounding his depression.

Based on my initial clinical impression, I knew I had to go slow and build trust before we could address specific issues. So for the next few sessions, we spent more time gathering background information and getting a feel for his strengths and weaknesses. Because he was shy and withdrawn, this process took time. What surprised me was that he wanted to return for further outpatient visits. Over the next few months, I could observe an emotional shift of being more open and willing to discuss personal issues including his pain. At this time, I had started a pain support group based on an educational and problem-solving model. I was pleasantly surprised when the patient expressed a desire to join.

After a couple of months in therapy, he described what sounded like a panic attack and he made the association that anxiety increased his pain level. This is what I consider a teachable moment! We spent some time on how our emotions can affect the perception of pain. It took a while, but he was now appreciating the importance of understanding the mind-body connection. I also felt it was an appropriate time to introduce more educational background which included the pain management workbook that I mentioned previously and Herbert Benson's book, *The Relaxation Response*. I have used this reference for a number of years. It is well written, understandable and discusses in depth the mind-body connection. In addition, Benson uses controlling high blood pressure as a clinical example, which was of interest to the patient since he also experienced high blood pressure.

This experience led to another teachable moment. I explained about the role that the sympathetic nervous system plays with both blood pressure and the perception of pain. He shared with me that his wife monitored his blood pressure (BP) on a daily basis. In his case, it was very helpful to be married to a nurse. I asked him if he would chart his BP on a piece of graph paper as well as his pain level at the same time as his wife was taking his BP. He was open to this task so he started collecting data. Further, I asked him to draw lines from day to day on both his BP and pain level and keep it public, where the family could see it. This was a big step for him as he is a very private person with a strong self-perceived masculine persona.

As I mentioned earlier, keeping track of behaviors (self-monitoring) is a powerful therapeutic tool, and keeping it public adds more power or self-reinforcing information that can ultimately change behavior.

I became interested in this connection during my doctoral graduate training which resulted in a lengthy doctoral dissertation that is still available online for those of you who are not familiar with this research. Subsequently, in each follow-up session, he produced more data for discussion, which opened the door to how he could control his sympathetic reactivity through relaxation training augmented by biofeedback.

For the next six months, I saw the patient individually and in a group setting. The group was beneficial for the patient because he could observe other pain patients talk about their pain and hear suggestions from group members how to problem solve.

I think over time he felt more comfortable with the group setting although he was never very talkative. I could tell he was actively listening and benefiting from hearing what others in the group had to say. My approach to group pain management was a combination of education, problem-solving and emotional support.

Group experiences are not appropriate for every pain patient; therefore, the provider needs to use discretion when selecting patients to join a group. Pain patients as a whole are very private and are not comfortable in a group setting. This patient was the exception since he was a private individual, but he was also very open and wanted to learn more about pain.

Unfortunately, during this period he experienced a number of health issues. Seizure activity reappeared, which resulted in visiting a neurosurgeon who requested an MRI. His neurosurgeon suggested adding Baclofen at bedtime, which appeared to help his sleep and seizure activity. Additionally, financial stress was taking a toll and he started to worry that he may lose his home. His PCP was performing trigger point injections (TPI) in the head and neck region that were helpful, especially in conjunction with physical therapy. At this time, we also received the results of his sleep study. As we suspected, he was diagnosed with central sleep apnea. He tried a CPAP but found it uncomfortable and therefore refused to wear any kind of breathing device.

He continued to come to group and invited his wife to join him, which I interpreted as a positive indication since she was his primary care giver. We also continued with individual sessions that were mainly focused on monitoring, problem-solving, and emotional support. We would also spend part of the session practicing his relaxation skills. His pain levels were trending downward, around 4/10 for an average. He was more active than previously, continuing his pool therapy, and his affect or mood improved. He also wanted to cut back on his opioid pain medicines since he felt they were compromising his memory. We adjusted his hydrocodone from 4–6 per day to 3 per day. In addition, his PCP adjusted back his Duragesic patch. He reported improvement in his memory and energy level.

By now we were in the third year of treatment. The group had finished and I was now seeing him monthly, primarily for maintenance and occasional problem-solving. He was satisfied with this schedule since he was paying more out-of-pocket, so seeing him fewer times reduced his financial burden. We had been working on his smoking over the past year and he was down to 10 cigarettes/day, which I considered a major achievement. I use a basic behavioral approach to smoking management. I had the patient carry an ashtray with him everywhere he went, including driving in the car. At the end of the day, I had him count his butts and add this number to his chart. Research has suggested that this simple act of self-monitoring will cut smoking by a third.

We kept progressing over the next few years, especially in improved coping with family stressors. His sister moved out, which improved the home environment. He was then able to use his basement again as his private space. Financial issues continued to increase, which was taking a toll on him. His pain management physician was concerned about tolerance to his opioid pain medicines. He suggested a spinal trial to determine if the patent would be an appropriate candidate for an implantable infusion pump. This was not an unusual option considering the patient had been taking oral opioid-based medicines for years. One of the advantages of a pump is that you can achieve therapeutic levels of opioid pain medicines at a fraction of the oral dose. This is also an advantage as it is easier on the end-organs over the long haul.

The implant surgery went well, but as I warned the patient, there is always a painful ramp-up period until the optimal level is achieved. At first, the pump was providing only about 30% pain coverage. It took several months to adjust the pump up to a therapeutic level. His pain management physician started with a combination of morphine plus Clonadine, which had a positive secondary affect of lowering his blood pressure. His pain control improved, his mood improved, and he complained less about cognitive side effects. As his pain improved he became more active. One of his favorite pastimes was feeding the squirrels in his backyard. Pump maintenance is a complicated process that takes constant care and adjustments. After a couple of years, his pain physician changed his morphine to Dilaudid, based on GI complaints by the patient. Over time, this change appeared beneficial since his GI complaints subsided and his pain levels stabilized.

I continued to see this patient over the next few years on a PRN basis. Looking back, his overall quality of life had improved, he continued to use his behavioral techniques, and his PCP felt he was more compliant with treatment. While neither his life nor his pain control were perfect, he was happier and enjoyed life more. In a complex case like this, the provider needs to keep expectations realistic and flexible. For me, it was a real life lesson of patience. As I look back, it was valuable for me to be involved with this patient, since I had the skills and took the time to stick with him, even though at times it looked hopeless.

Unfortunately, my last contact with him was a legal notice from the bankruptcy court asking me if I would write off his outstanding bill. I heard that by filing for bankruptcy, he was able to keep his home. I was happy to do so since I had learned a great deal from this patient.

Patient #4

This is an interesting case worthy of our discussion for a number of reasons. First, he presented with an unusual pain condition. Second, there were protracted and very adversarial legal issues that included a number of Independent Medical Evaluations (IME). Third, according to my records, he saw over 20 physicians with various specialties over the course of his medical treatment, which lasted sixteen years. Because of the scope and length of this care, I will condense our discussion to the pertinent facts.

Psychosocial Background

He was born and raised in southern California. He reported no problems in public school stating that he was a good student who was active in sports. There was no reported history of abuse, no drug or alcohol problems, and no remarkable early health issues. After high school, he entered the plumbing trade working his way up to journeyman plumber. While working in Hawaii as a plumber, he experienced a significant work injury when he was run over by a truck.

Since this case involves a diagnosis of Chronic Regional Pain Syndrome (CRPS) I am going to include a brief introduction to this diagnosis. There are considerable disagreements within the field of pain medicine regarding CRPS due to the lack of animal models and precise testing methods. There are two accepted types of CRPS. Type I may develop after trauma but with no objective nerve lesion findings. Type II develops after trauma with objectively assessed nerve lesions. An extreme view of CRPS I is thought to be more of a psychiatric condition (somatoform) but is now generally disregarded. It is important to note that the leading national proponent of this thinking is a prominent neurologist from Portland, Oregon, who evaluated this patient.

Generally, it is believed that CRPS patients show sympathetic, somato-motor and somato-sensory contributions, and it is believed to be primarily an inflammatory disease in the extremities as a consequence of nerve damage. It is believed that there are central mechanisms and autonomic systems that are triggered by peripheral input. The bottom line is that CRPS is not well understood, there is little empirical data and there is no accepted treatment protocol that produces consistent results. This disagreement within pain medicine directly relates to my earlier comments regarding the impact of Cartesian dualistic thinking or the either/or school of thinking. It is either psychogenic in origin, that is Type I or Type II, which demonstrates objective damage to the nerves (sensory). This patient got caught in this controversy, which influenced the treatment he received.

Medical History

I will summarize the main findings and treatments he received over the past ten years that relate directly to my above conclusions. As stated above, he received an injury to his spine while working. He was first treated by a chiropractor, who diagnosed thoracic lumbar and cervical strains, which fits within the scope of chiropractic care. He then underwent a CT scan of the lumbar spine that was essentially negative and surgery was ruled out. He was then treated by a board-certified pain medicine specialist who released the patient to return to work.

A few months later, the patient sought out a surgical consult, which included an MRI scan that showed moderate central disc herniation at L5-S1. He then underwent an anterior fusion surgery, which resulted in a burning sensation in both his legs. His left foot became cold and sensitive to touch, which prompted the surgeon to hypothesize that the patient may have CRPS. He then underwent a series of lumbar sympathetic blocks with no relief.

At this point, two years after his initial injury, he was implanted with a spinal cord stimulator, which produced some pain relief. He was then evaluated by another surgeon who performed a left lumbar sympathectomy, which resulted in increased warmth to his foot but also an increase in pain.

Because of continued pain, he was then referred for another neurosurgical evaluation who diagnosed the patient's condition as a left L4-5 radiculopathy secondary to lumbar spinal stenosis and disc disease, reflex sympathetic dystrophy (CRPS) of the left leg. The neurosurgeon then recommended a discogram and decompressive spine surgery. The discogram showed mild bulging of the L4-5 disc without focal herniation. Remember that an earlier MRI indicated a moderate disc herniation at L5-S1. I would like to emphasize that the inconsistency in "objective" testing contributed to the ongoing surgical interventions. Also keep in mind, during the first five years of surgical treatment, the patient was never referred for a psychological consultation.

The patient's pain persisted which resulted in another surgery, this time a decompressive bilateral laminectomy and foraminotomies at the L5-S1 level. The patient reported no pain relief after this surgery. With little or no pain relief, the patient was considered for an intrathecal pump. After a successful spinal trial, he received the permanent pump, which provided moderate pain relief.

Approximately six months after the placement of the pump, the patient reported severe pain in the left leg, low back, left arm, and head. His primary surgeon then stated that the patient's reflex sympathetic dystrophy condition had progressed and he noted the patient's left hand was dark red, cold, and painful to touch. The following year the patient underwent another evaluation, which concluded that the patient should undergo a psychiatric evaluation to assess the patient's suspected depression. This same physician also recommended that the patient should relocate to an area that offered a multidisciplinary pain program. This recommendation resulted in the patient moving to the Bay Area where he was evaluated by a prominent pain physician who diagnosed the patient with persistent low back pain with bilateral leg pain, functional thoracic outlet syndrome, and diffuse muscle pain. It is interesting to note that he did not comment on the patient's previous diagnosis of RSD or CRPS. This evaluation recommended intravenous Lidocaine infusions, a trial of Keppra, Topanox, and physical therapy.

Based on the forgoing recommendations, the patient then moved to Portland, Oregon, where he was evaluated by the OHSU pain management program. His spinal cord stimulator was revised and according to his records from OHSU, his spinal stimulator was providing relief for the lower extremity but not for the low back. The patient then transferred his care to a pain management physician in private practice who subsequently referred the patient to me for a psychological evaluation and therapy.

My initial clinical impression was that the patient had a very complex medical history that included numerous surgical interventions, including implantable pain technology. Most of his pain was in the low back, with additional pain in his hands and feet, which were cold to touch and blue in color. He rated his pain at 6/10, with a low of 4/10 to a high of 9/10. He continued his prescription from Hawaii, which consisted orally of 4 Ultracet plus his Oxycodone. This was in addition to his infusion pump, which provided a combination of morphine and Clonadine. He estimated that he received 50% pain relief from both his infusion pump and his spinal cord stimulator, but received no pain relief in his hands.

The patient reported he was married for the second time with no children. He further related he was not close to his parents or his two brothers. He denied any previous psychiatric history and stated prior to his injury he was active and led a normal life. He related to me in a pleasant forth-coming manner with no obvious psychosocial distress. He was not confused and exhibited excellent memory, but his affect suggested that he was sad, primarily over his inability to work and provide for his family.

I suggested a trial course of biofeedback with a focus on temperature feedback. He was open to this suggestion and I also included information on mind/body medicine. We started with basic progressive relaxation with time for supportive talk. He progressed well and we quickly moved into autogenic therapy with excellent results. He was practicing at home on a daily basis and his peripheral skin temperatures were improving. This was a surprising outcome considering his previous sympathectomy. I suspected his sympathectomy was incomplete or that his nerves had reconnected which resulted in warmer extremities. At this point in therapy, I could tell he was becoming more open and trusting so I introduced vocational counseling and we discussed possible training and jobs that would be appropriate based on his condition.

After four sessions, I invited his wife to sit in with us. She provided additional valuable information. The patient was presenting a personal picture of emotional strength and downplaying any psychosocial distress associated with his pain. According to his wife's account, the patient was depressed and not sleeping well. I then added an additional component to therapy, which involved a cognitive behavioral approach to treat his depression. This addition was well received by both the patient and his wife. Further, his autogenic training was going well where he could raise his skin temperature from 84 degrees to 90 degrees after a 30 min exercise.

At this point in time, his workers' compensation program ordered two Independent Medical Evaluations (IME): One from a prominent local neurologist who I mentioned earlier, who specialized in nerve injury, and the other by a psychiatrist who was well known as a "hired gun." The neurological evaluation concluded that the only diagnosis related to the work injury were cervical, thoracic, and lumbar strain. They further concluded that the patient suffered from a "pseudo-neurological" pain disorder. He concluded that the pseudo-neurological pain disorder did not relate to any aspect of the original injury or to any direct effects of his surgical treatments. The neurologist then added that psychosocial factors were playing a strong role in perpetuating his current symptomatology. The only medical treatment recommended from this neurological IME was psychiatric treatment. This evaluator also stated that the patient did not require any work restrictions based on their findings.

What this evaluation is implying is that the patient is experiencing conversion hysteria and that he is malingering. I remember when I first read this report I could not believe what I was seeing, and it was far from the facts that were well documented. They had completely distorted what was known about this patient and his history. First, I have to admit that I know this neurologist quite well and I have testified in court on other cases that he had evaluated. The patient had no psychiatric history prior to his work injury. According to his wife, he had a long productive work history and he enjoyed being a journeyman plumber. All of his psychological symptoms started after his work injury and were compounded by repeated surgical failures.

His psychiatric IME literally added "insult to injury." The psychiatrist relied heavily on the results of a psychological test called the Minnesota Multiphasic Personality Inventory (MMPI) to formulate his conclusions. I am very familiar with this test, since I attended the University of Minnesota where this test was developed. I have administered this test to over 5,000 pain patients and I know its strengths and weaknesses. Further, the psychiatrist who conducted the IME relied on a "canned" actuarial interpretation, which is based on cut-off scores. In addition, the test is premised on purely dualistic thinking on which I have already commented. Based on how the test was constructed and how the computer interprets the responses to the questions predetermines the profile the patient will exhibit. Because I have received extensive training with this instrument, I know how to interpret the results and I do not rely on the "canned" interpretation. It was obvious to me the psychiatrist in question had no idea what the results were showing since the computer also provides the diagnosis of somatoform pain disorder, which implies conversion hysteria and was consistent with the earlier neurological IME. I will not get into a detailed discussion or critique of the MMPI construct validity issues, especially when it is administered to any patient with a chronic health condition. The patient's demonstrated elevated anxiety level or sympathetic reactivity can also elevate the hysteria scale, which the computer program cannot determine. Finally, to top it all off, the psychiatrist concluded that the patient's somatoform disorder was not caused by his work injury. The patient was being totally discredited based on thinking that goes back to the 17th century. I should add that the psychiatrist spent a total of 45 minutes talking to this patient!

I wrote numerous letters to his workers' compensation carrier and their attorneys arguing that the two IMEs were misleading and a distortion of the facts. My argument was that the patient was anxious and depressed based not only on his work injury, but also on repeated surgical interventions, which only compounded his suffering. He was not making up his symptoms! I felt it was a grievous insult, not only to the patient, but also to both the professions of neurology and psychiatry.

The patient won his case based on medical evidence.

Summary

The patient did well for me; he worked hard in regaining some personal control over his body and both his mood and sleep improved. After about a year of seeing this patient and his wife in therapy, they decided to move to southern California where they both had family and the climate would be more conducive to his continued mental and physical health.

The value of including this case for discussion is hopefully clear to the reader. The patient saw too many doctors all of whom wanted to help but were surgeons using the "I can fix it model" without considering a multidisciplinary approach and without a deep understanding of the nature of pain. There was no consideration of the patient as a holistic organism, but only of his parts. In hindsight, one wonders if the patient had not had that first surgery, what would have been the course of his pain and his pain treatment?

All too often we do not trust our bodies to heal themselves even though they have been doing so for over a million years. We become impatient and want results immediately and can become our own worst enemy. It should be obvious to the reader that the many repeated surgical interventions this patient experienced added more scar tissue, which can be a pain generator in itself. Further, repeated surgical failures added to a sense of despondency, which was directly related to his work injury. He trusted his medical providers to help him, but in the end they became part of the problem and not the solution. This is where the role of common sense comes into play.

Patient #5

I wanted to include this patient for discussion since he presented with a very unique and rare pain experience. He was very pleasant and easy to work with. There was no confusion. He was very verbal and there were no secondary gain issues.

He was single, had never married, and had no children. His parents were deceased, he had no siblings and admitted to having very few friends. He was living in a Catholic care facility, which was stressful, since he enjoyed smoking cigars.

His formal education ended at high school, although I estimated that he was in the average range of intelligence. He enjoyed school, was not active in sports and admitted no learning problems, and no drug or alcohol abuse. There was no history of psychological issues with him or in his family. He stated he had very few friends in school and for the most part was socially isolated which was also the case as an adult. He did not appear to be overtly anxious or depressed, which was confirmed by repeated testing that was required by his health insurance company. At times he was frustrated with his health care, which was with a large Catholic-managed health care organization. He never became angry and overall maintained a positive mental outlook.

He had worked for the railroad loading and unloading boxcars. He reportedly enjoyed his work and indicated that it was not stressful. However, one day while he was working, he slipped and fell under a moving boxcar, which resulted in a traumatic amputation of his left leg, just above his knee. He was referred to me for behavioral treatment of his stump and phantom pain issues. At the time of my initial evaluation he was in his mid-50s, in good health with the exception of elevated blood pressure, which was controlled well with medicine.

He was referred to me by his pain physician, who I knew well. He had undergone a number of injections, which provided little or no relief. My initial impression was that he was open to behavioral treatment.

At the time I started treating this patient, a very good book on phantom pain was published by Richard Sherman, PhD. Dr. Sherman was an Army psychologist who specialized in phantom pain which was prevalent in the Army post-Vietnam era. He conducted an extensive survey of 11,000 veterans and found that 80% reported significant phantom pain. Keep in mind that his sample was entirely of cases of traumatic amputation, which was consistent with the patient we are now discussing.

Phantom pain is difficult to understand; how could a patient describe pain in a limb that was no longer there? Consequently, many amputees are afraid to discuss their phantom pain for fear of losing credibility, since it must be "all in their head." This was discussed in both Chapters 1 and 2 of this book. Dualistic thinking is still evident in medicine, especially when considering how a patient could experience phantom pain.

Sherman also found in his survey that there was no association of pre-amputation pain and post-amputation pain (phantom and stump). This was also true of this patient. He had no premorbid history of chronic pain, nor did his family. Research in the 80s and 90s by Marshall Devore, Richard Sherman, Joel Katz, Ron Melzack and others led to the assumption that amputation does not silence afferent nerve signals from the limb. In fact, it may augment the signal. We now know that the proximal stump of severed nerves and associated dorsal root ganglia generate ectopic spontaneous and evoked discharge that gives rise to sensation referred to the missing limb (phantom limb). Further, it is now assumed that amplification processes within the CNS may augment the phantom signal and distort it. Unfortunately, surgical procedures have not produced therapeutic solutions. It is also interesting to note that Joel Katz found that pain memories are precise sensations, indistinguishable from pains experienced before amputation.

In their research, Joel Katz and Ron Melzack did not find any differences in depression, anxiety, or personality characteristics between a sample of amputees with phantom pain and a matched sample of pain-free peers. Reassessment after five years confirmed the above findings. The role of psycho-physiological arousal or sympathetic reactivity has also been examined. A review by Sherman found that both stump and phantom pain are affected by stress, which is also true of other pain syndromes. This patient was consistent with the above conclusions in that he described higher pain ratings in both his stump and phantom pain when he became frustrated with his insurance carrier.

I saw this patient for 40 individual sessions over a period of three years. The initial phase of treatment focused on the basics of pain management, building trust and history. As I mentioned earlier, he was open and motivated to pursue behavioral treatment, especially since he experienced little or no relief with injection therapy.

When I asked him to describe his phantom pain he used graphic adjectives such as gripping, throbbing, and burning. When his pain level was the highest, he described his phantom toes curling which set off a spasm in his phantom foot. It is interesting to note that he also described stump pain, which for the most part covaried with his phantom pain. This association between the two pains is also consistent in the research literature.

One of his main frustrations was his perception that his prosthetic leg did not fit well and his insurance carrier would not approve a new leg. My visual inspection of his stump confirmed his account that the end of the stump was inflamed, hot to the touch and highly sensitive. Because of these issues he rarely wore his prosthetic leg. I contacted his primary care physician (PCP) and his surgeon to express my concerns that the patient needed to be reevaluated for a new leg. His mobility and quality of life were compromised by a poor fitting prosthetic leg. Further, 50% of the patient's pain was stump pain and if the research is correct, stump pain is directly associated with phantom pain. It took over a year of advocating for a new leg before he was fitted for a new state of the art prosthetic leg. The new leg contributed to a significant pain reduction in both the stump and phantom pains. He dropped from 6/10 to 3/10, his mood improved and he was more mobile.

Initially, his pain physician prescribed 30mg of MS Contin, which according to the patient was helpful. The research suggests that both stump and phantom pain should be considered forms of neuropathic pain. When I was part of the OHSU pain management team we were conducting research on the utilization of Neurontin for neuropathic pain. At that time it was considered off label since it was only approved for seizure control. I contacted his pain physician suggesting a trial of Neurontin starting at a low dose, increasing his dose while monitoring for negative side effects. The primary negative side effect of Neurontin is dizziness. We worked him up to about 2000mg with significant pain relief in both the stump and phantom limb. Further, his pain physician prescribed a low dose TCA at bedtime which helped with sleep and pain control. As I mentioned in Chapter 4, there is a body of older research supporting the use of TCA antidepressant medication that contributes to improved pain control.

After we established a basis of trust, I introduced relaxation therapy augmented by biofeedback. I focused on temperature feedback since it is a valid and reliable indication of sympathetic arousal. I monitored the temperature, with a surface thermistor on his intact limb. Temperature readings from his intact foot were in the normal ranges of high 80s to low 90s. It is interesting to note that when he described his phantom limb it was always cold. I then initiated a plan to approach both his intact limb and his phantom limb. First, we focused on his intact limb with progressive relaxation techniques (tense/relax) plus deep breathing. When he could raise the skin temperature in his intact foot he reported his phantom foot also relaxed and it felt warmer. We then used autogenic therapy, which utilizes self phrasing of heavy and warm. I also added a visualization exercise where I would have him visualize his phantom limb when he repeated to himself that his leg was heavy and warm. Using both of these techniques together appeared to have a synergistic effect, which resulted in lower pain in both the stump and phantom limb. It is important to note that he was doing this by himself, to himself, which gave him a sense of control over his pain. This is a very strong self-reinforcing process that counteracts feelings of helplessness and hopelessness, the two main ingredients in what we call depression, which is a common phenomenon with all pain patients.

The final phase of therapy, which occurred in the third year was maintenance. Maintenance is of value when the patient is willing and motivated to come in on a monthly basis for regular maintenance since it will prevent relapse. This patient was highly motivated because he experienced success, which was highly reinforcing. His pain levels in both the stump and phantom limb dropped over 50%, which he attributed to his new leg and the effectiveness of behavioral therapy which gave him more personal control of the pain. The quality of his life also improved, which was due to increased mobility with lower, more manageable pain levels.

Before he lost his leg he was an avid motorcycle rider. When he lost his leg he had to sell his motorcycle, which was very sad for him. Now he started thinking he wanted to ride again and fulfill a lifelong dream of riding his motorcycle to the annual Sturgis, SD, motorcycle festival. I suggested he might want to try out a three wheel motorcycle for safety reasons. He was open to that suggestion. My last contact with him was a postcard from Sturgis, SD, telling me he was having a great time.

Patient #6

This patient presents a complicated medical and psychosocial history. His pain started after a horrific accident that almost ended his life. He is still on my active caseload. He was referred by his attorney who specializes in representing workers' compensation cases. This attorney is exceptional in that he cares about his client's total welfare, which I appreciate as an allied health provider.

The original date of injury was in 2011 and my initial involvement was one year later. The first year after the accident was occupied by multiple surgeries and getting the patient medically stable. At the time of the accident he was working as a supervisor for an oil-drilling firm in Texas. According to the patient and his initial ER records, he was working on a drilling rig platform, pressure testing holes when a pipe burst underneath him propelling him some 30 feet in the air.

His preoperative diagnosis was left mid-foot fracture-dislocation with fracture of the medial, middle and lateral cuneiforms as well as the cuboid and the base of the second, third and fourth metatarsals, plus gross dislocation of the first, second, third, fourth and fifth tarsometatarsal joints. He was life-flighted to a hospital where he underwent extensive surgery. He was unconscious at the time of his transport but regained consciousness by the time he arrived at the ER. There was serious thought he would lose his left limb but he would not consent. He also experienced severe head trauma, which required numerous sutures, but no fractures. A post-operative CT of his head revealed soft tissue swelling/hematoma along posterior right parietal area of his head. CT scans of his chest and spine were unremarkable.

After two weeks in intensive care in Texas, he was transferred by air ambulance to a large hospital in Portland. A complete evaluation was performed using CT scans of both his lower left extremity and head. The results indicated that orthopedic hardware had not changed position, his fractures were also unchanged, and his head CT indicated no acute intracranial hemorrhage. After one month in the hospital in Portland, the patient underwent additional surgery that included removal of the external fixator on his left foot and multiple plate fixations with screws. One month later, a third surgery was performed where additional fixations were completed. In addition, a deep left calf vein thrombosis was diagnosed and he was placed on Coumadin. He was also referred for PT and rehabilitation. At the time he became an outpatient, he was prescribed oxycodone, 15mg x2/day, plus one 5mg, Bacofen 10mg/day, Tylenol 500mg PRN/, Lyrica 100mg, and Coumadin 5mg. In early 2012, his fourth surgery was performed to remove his hardware. At this point, the patient was experiencing recurrent pain in his left leg and foot in the range of 5/10 while undergoing physical therapy in and out of the pool.

Approximately one year after his accident, he underwent his first Independent Medical Examination (IME). At this time he described his pain as sharp and then a dull ache. He also described pinpoint needles-type sensation at times. Any type of pressure on his foot, including walking, produced a hot sensation that shifted to cold. He also noted discoloration in his foot and that his toenails were becoming soft. He reported pain at night, which disrupted his sleep. This IME was performed by a podiatrist who diagnosed the patient with post-traumatic mid foot fracture and chronic regional pain syndrome, Type I. The evaluator justified the diagnosis of CRPS I by noting the following symptoms: hyperalgesia, allodynia, edema, temperature changes, plus tropic skin changes. This diagnosis was confirmed at the same IME by a neurologist who noted that the CRPS I diagnosis was reasonable and definite. It is important to point this out since at a later IME, the CRPS diagnosis was questioned. Both reviewers believed the patient to be believable and straightforward, with the recommendation that he be treated from a multidisciplinary pain management program.

One year after his accident, he was referred to me by his attorney who specializes in workers' compensation cases. I had worked with this attorney on previous cases and found him to be a compassionate individual who cared about the wellbeing of his clients.

The patient was being cared for by a primary care physician who was approved by his workers' compensation carrier. He was prescribed 10mg of Oxycodone 1/day at bedtime, but received no relief. He tried hydrocodone but it upset his stomach so it was discontinued. He rated his pain as 7/10 with a low of 4/10 to a high of 10/10 at night. He described his number one pain in his left foot that radiated up into his leg. He further described his pain similar to electric shock that was associated with movement and was hypersensitive to touch and extreme weather. His number two pain he associated with his low back and rated this pain at 3/10 with a high of 8/10. He described this pain as a constant ache that is worse with activity and no radiating pain into his legs. His number three pain was headaches with some pain in his right jaw which he associated with clenching. Remember that he was diagnosed with a concussion as a result of his accident. He related that he had no previous history of headaches.

His early health history revealed experimenting with drugs and alcohol. It should also be noted that there was an extensive history of alcohol abuse in his family and he did admit that he was physically abused by his father. He admitted that he does not like to take drugs for his pain, but will smoke marijuana, which helps to relax him. His home life could be described as stressful, since he is the primary caretaker for his mother who is disabled. At this time, his girlfriend was also living with him and she also had significant medical issues.

After an extended evaluation of this patient I concurred with his previous IME, that the patient was experiencing significant pain on a recurrent basis due in part to his nerve damage that was part of his CRPS Type I. Further, he was extremely anxious with a history of panic that compounded his pain. His low back and head pain were also compounded by his elevated anxiety level, which resulted in increased muscle tension. I also noted that he might qualify for an additional diagnosis of Post-Traumatic Stress Disorder (PTSD) as a result of his accident. In addition, I documented that his sleep disorder (insomnia) existed as a result of his accident and subsequent recurrent pain.

His formal schooling was sporadic. He did not finish high school nor did he complete his GED, although he did attend community college for three to four semesters and completed a certificate program in business management. My initial impression was that he was bright, or above average intellectually, and that he was curious to obtain new information. My impression was also that he was open to returning to school to learn an occupation that was not physically demanding. His work history suggested that he was an achiever, as reflected by the job he had when he was injured. He had worked up to a supervisor position and was earning $12,000 a month. He was saving his money, plus supporting his mother, sister, and a son, aged 10, from a previous relationship. He was receiving $4,000 a month from his workers' compensation carrier and he related that he was under constant financial pressure.

Because of his fragile nature, I spent considerable time in supportive psychotherapy early in our relationship. I needed to build his trust in me to form the basis for a more proactive approach to his pain management. Once he was psychologically stable, I considered a referral to a comprehensive rehabilitation program. Because it would require him to be gone for 28 days, he objected, stating that it would be too hard on his family for him to be absent for that length of time. I also referred him to a pain management physician, who altered his pain medicine and switched him from morphine to methadone and increased his Effexor to 75mg.

He mentioned that the methadone was helpful and there was no itching, which he experienced with the morphine. He was also scheduled for a series of nerve blocks. Unfortunately, the initial nerve block did not go well and he declined further injections. His pain levels during this period remained at approximately the same level around 7/10 in his foot and 4/10 in his back, but they were less labile, which I interpreted as a positive initial trend.

One of the many stressors that influenced my treatment was transportation. Many days he would not show for his appointment because he could not find a ride. I spoke with his attorney about this issue and we decided to appeal to his workers' compensation carrier to provide transportation. After numerous letters, his carrier agreed to the request, which improved treatment compliance, which had a secondary effect of improving his mental outlook. He looked forward to our meetings and felt they were helpful. During this period, his workers' compensation carrier assigned a vocational counselor to work on retraining plans. At first, I thought it was premature since his pain levels and the amount of psychosocial distress he was experiencing would undermine any immediate vocational plans. As I found out later, once a vocational plan has been formulated, a rigid timeline for completion is imposed and the vocational counselor is not paid if the timeline is not met. This condition imposed additional stress on the patient, since the vocational counselor had his own agenda independent of his clinical treatment. After consulting with the patient's attorney we agreed that at this time vocational planning was inappropriate, especially since this counselor was very insistent about meeting the timeline goals. After protracted negotiation with his carrier, vocational counseling was suspended for the present.

The focus of our treatment during this middle period was devoted to emotional support, problem-solving from a cognitive behavioral perspective, and stress management. It was a difficult period for the patient because of the number of stressors that would occur unexpectedly. His live-in girlfriend's health status was not good. She required numerous emergency hospitalizations. His mother's health was deteriorating, and his sister was a constant worry because of her drug issues. On top of all of this, he continued to have significant financial pressure.

Keep in mind that stress is additive and accumulates over time. The stress had a direct impact on his nervous system (sympathetic reactivity) that in turn influenced his pain. In a reciprocal fashion, his increased pain then negatively impacted his ability to cope, which added more stress. The experience was like trying to plug a hole, but with a new hole to plug each week.

At this time, his carrier assigned a new primary care physician (PCP) to oversee his medical care. Unfortunately, this individual was not a pain physician, but a general care physician who was not supportive of pain medicine or psychotropics. Also during this period, his girlfriend's parents decided to move their daughter back home, since her health was not improving. This had both a positive and a negative impact on the patient since he would not be able to see her as they lived 300 miles away. He cared deeply for her and this was a significant emotional loss for him. The positive effect was that it removed a daily stressor that had a significant impact on the patient's wellbeing. He now had more time to focus on his own treatment and rehabilitation.

My therapy approach with this patient was split approximately 50/50. Half of the time was supportive, since he was still very emotional about what was going on in his life. The other half was more instructive from a cognitive behavioral approach, especially helping him reframe negative, worrying thoughts. He remained open and motivated which was helpful, but I still felt that there were so many holes to plug! He gave me permission to talk to his new PCP, which I did. I shared some of my thoughts regarding his treatment and he was open to a psychotropic medicine to help moderate his anxiety level. The PCP did prescribe Elavil, 25mg h.s. and Xanax, 1mg PRN, which gave the patient some relief in both anxiety and pain. The patient did not want to try a GABA medicine since he had had a bad experience with Neurontin and he wanted to stay away from opioid-based pain medicines.

After a couple of weeks, he reported that both medicines were helpful especially with promoting more sleep. He only took his Xanax sparingly since we discussed the potential for abuse. We started working on basic problems of living including setting up a budget and what he can do to prepare for school. I gave him some homework exercises that included going out to a school and scheduling an appointment with a counselor. These exercises were based on a desensitization model since he was anxious about returning to school. However, he was experiencing fewer panic attacks, down from daily to 1 or 2 a week. He felt the relaxation skills plus the Xanax were helpful. In addition, I instructed him to monitor the skin temperature in both feet, with the right foot being the control and his left (injured) foot, which was cooler, being the experimental variable. By this time, we were using both progressive relaxation techniques and autogenics with both visualization and self-phrasing. "My foot is heavy and warm." His goal was to increase the skin temperature on the left foot to approximate the skin temperature of his right or "control" foot. I have used adhesive skin thermistors for years and find them very useful and reliable. Patients can take them home for practice in their own environment.

Upon my return from vacation, the patient reported that he did complete his homework, and in my estimation, exceeded it! He spent two weeks exploring the campus and he spoke to a counselor. He found out that he needed to take a math class to meet the prerequisites for the program he was interested in. They assured him that they would provide tutors through the learning lab, and a peer tutor if necessary. The next step was to propose a plan to his workers' compensation carrier and his vocational counselor. My approach to this issue was to get the patient involved, to make it his plan, and not the plan of an independent vocational counselor who had a different agenda. We had to start this plan early since it had to go through an approval process with both the college and his workers' compensation carrier. We set the goal to start in the fall, and it was April at the time, so it would be close.

The next phase of therapy focused on stress and pain control, with the addition of vocational counseling and preparing for school. His pain levels were more stable during this period and he was successfully coping with all the stressors in his life. He was more active outside, working in his yard and walking since the weather was improving. He had a meeting with his attorney who was not optimistic that his workers' compensation carrier would approve his educational plan.

At this time he was assigned a new vocational counselor who was more positive and involved. She felt he would do well in a construction management program that would last two years. Since he had fifteen years of experience in construction, she assumed it would be a good fit. The patient had other ideas. He felt more interested in the mechatronics program with construction management as a backup plan. Also at this time, he went through a physical capacity examination.

We were pleasantly surprised when we found out that his educational plan was approved by his workers' compensation carrier. This set up a new challenge since the patient's anxiety level increased with the thought of starting school in the fall. From a therapeutic perspective, we now started working on more desensitization, pairing the relaxation response with visualization involving school situations.

Medically, he met with his primary care physician, who increased his Elavil to 50mg h.s. The patient reported more dry mouth and more GI distress as a result. He was also taking Xanax on a more regular basis to counteract his increasing frequency of panic. I noted no cognitive issues or confusion after both of these increases. He registered for fall classes and he was optimistic.

The patient completed a battery of aptitude tests, which indicated that he was high functioning in all areas except math. Mentally he was improving and his gait also improved even though he continued to use his cane for balance. He demonstrated initiative by buying his math book early and was using the tutor center before the start of classes. His sleep remained an issue even though he was taking his Elavil at bedtime. My own thinking at that time was his level of arousal was increased due to the start of school.

I had a number of concerns about his ability to cope with school, including extensive walking between classes, prolonged sitting time at a desk, and continuing transportation challenges. Therapeutically, we continued to work on stress management, using his relaxation skills before class and tests. At midterms, he reported that he was doing well except for math, which continued to be a challenge. He mentioned that he was going to the tutor center for extra help and he had not missed one class.

He continued to work hard throughout the second half of the semester, achieving high grades in all his classes, including math. He was staying active and was not complaining about his foot pain or his sleep problems.

He continued to learn new relaxation techniques, including extending his autogenics into self-hypnosis. His biofeedback readings also improved as indicated by a 10 degree increase after 30 minutes of practice in the office. He was also using his relaxation techniques at school and at home, which was a positive sign of his motivation to succeed in his chosen activities. His final exams went well and he earned 2 A's, 1 B, and 1 C, which he could not understand. Overall, his performance was outstanding to my way of thinking, especially when you consider all the hurdles he had overcome. Further, it gave him confidence he could do well in school and he looked forward to his second semester.

During winter break, the patient came down with a nasty viral bug that laid him up for weeks. He missed a number of classes at the beginning of the term, which contributed to his anxiety level, which was already high. To complicate matters, he was involved in a serious auto accident that resulted in his car being totaled. This added more anxiety and caused him to be without transportation so he could not get to school. Naturally, his workers' compensation carrier did not look positively on this, especially missing classes. His vocational counselor became concerned and put more pressure on the patient since she had a timeline to meet. The result was the patient retreated and stayed at home, not returning phone calls from his attorney, vocational counselor, or myself. This was not good for him since it undermined his workers' compensation (insurance) carrier's confidence that he was on the right track to full rehabilitation. I had advised everyone involved that we were asking too much and that we should back off and give him some room. His school was supportive and suggested he take incompletes and focus on returning next fall. His attorney and I agreed that this was a reasonable plan. His vocational counselor and his insurance carrier were not so sure. They wanted to terminate the vocational plan and cash him out. It was now spring and we were at a stalemate. Both his attorney and I wrote a number of letters supporting the patient, pointing out how well he did his first semester.

Then a disaster occurred. His sister committed suicide in his home by hanging herself in his son's bedroom. This was the straw that broke the camel's back. He retreated further, shutting himself off from any outside contact. After a couple of weeks he agreed to come in for a talk. He was not in good shape. He blamed himself for not being more supportive. The focus of our therapy shifted to emotional support and working through his grief. After a month of intensive care that included many phone calls, he started to come around expressing a desire to return to school in the fall.

Of course his insurance carrier was losing patience, expressing doubts that he was able to return to school and perform to their standards. To make matters worse, they ordered an IME to be conducted by a psychiatrist. Keep in mind he had already gone through two previous IMEs that confirmed both his diagnoses and treatment plan. I have mentioned this point previously, but I felt that his insurance carrier was trying to stack the deck against the patient hoping for an adverse opinion so that they could close his case. IMEs are not independent in Oregon (contrary to the name). The IME reviewer is contracted by the insurance carrier, so there is an inherent conflict of interest since the reviewer wants to stay in the good graces of the insurance carrier and obtain more work. My fears were justified. It was the worst hatchet job I have ever read in my 40 years of practice. The examiner accused him of faking his symptoms and that his case has been a sham. Of course the patient was crushed and angry; I believe justifiably so, since the IME ignored his history and the many medical providers that had treated him over the past four years.

Consequently, his insurance carrier terminated my services since his IME reviewer concluded that he was ready to return to work, or in her words, he was medically stationary and he would not benefit from further treatment. She spent a total of 45 minutes with the patient face-to-face and based her conclusions on one brief evaluation. Naturally, both his attorney and I were appalled by this so-called independent evaluation.

We have initiated an appeals process that could take up to a year. I assured his attorney that I would testify personally at any hearing that is ordered. I had a long conversation with the patient informing him of my support for his case and urged him not to give up hope. I encouraged him to contact me at any time, day or night. The case is ongoing at this time. I am optimistic we will prevail.

Patient #7

This case is very special to me and is still on my active caseload. He has been my patient longer than any others and has been with me for about fifteen years. Having followed a patient for this amount of time provides valuable knowledge to me as a provider, which I want to share with other providers and fellow pain patients.

When I first evaluated this patient, I could not have predicted that he would still be on my active caseload 15 years later. He is not a passive-dependent personality type. He is quite the opposite, of a strong independent person who is very insightful and has a strong sense of self. He was referred to me by my former partner, a board certified pain physician, who felt I could provide psychological services on an ongoing basis.

His medical history was complex, with a work injury to his low back and a history of multiple surgeries. In fact, he was a patient to a well-known pain surgeon in Canada by the name of Dr. Kumar. Dr. Kumar was one of the first pain surgeons in North America to try spinal cord stimulation, and this patient was one of the first to undergo this procedure. Unfortunately, it did not go well, and greatly affected the patient for the rest of his life. He told me early in our relationship that he did not want to ever experience another surgery of any kind. I believed him, and this mindset opened the door to my services as an allied health provider.

I look for certain characteristics when I evaluate a patient to determine if they would be good candidates for supportive behavioral therapy:

- Patients need to possess enough intellectual strength to tackle new information.
- They must be motivated and participate as a full partner.
- They must be realistic and understand that we are not going to "cure" or "fix" their pain, but work to improve their quality of life.

In my initial estimation, he fit the criteria.

At the beginning, he reported his pain levels in the 5/10 range. I soon discovered that he was either under reporting his pain, or he was very stoic! He was athletic and had played hockey in Canada, so I assumed he had a high tolerance for pain. He was not aggressive or angry, which made it easier to work with him. He reported that he did not sleep well and I thought he might be depressed. His affect was not flat, nor was he self-destructive. I soon realized that his quiet manner was more of a personality trait and not an indication of any psychopathology. He was not overly trusting and it was uncomfortable for him to share personal information.

As I look back, it took over a year of knowing this patient before he would share information about himself. I let the patients decide if they want to share personal feelings. If they want to share, they will. I learned that he was married and he enjoyed his married life. He had no children, but he loved dogs and they had quite a few! His wife was strong and assertive. She did not feel shy about calling me and letting me know what I needed to do. Financially, they were comfortable with his disability payment and her salary. They lived on a rural property, which was ideal for raising dogs.

The other interesting aspect to this case was the amount of pain medicine he was taking. At first I was not so sure this was medically appropriate. Professionally I am not against pain medicine as long as the patient is carefully selected and monitored. Part of my job is to evaluate the patient for long-term opioid use. I feel that opioid pain medicine plays an important role in pain management and can be a useful tool, if the patient is carefully assessed by both a pain psychologist and the prescribing physician. This treatment should include a narcotic contract and periodic drug screens.

I reported back to the prescribing pain physician that in my estimation the patient was not drug seeking and that he was using his medicine appropriately. The use of opioid-based pain medicine is a hotly debated topic in my part of the country. I have been in this business long enough to experience fluctuations between support and opposition to opioid use. Currently, we are experiencing a negative swing based on an increasing frequency of opioid-related deaths. My own professional feelings are that patients are not being well-selected by a multidisciplinary team or monitored by a multidisciplinary team to avoid inappropriate prescriptions.

In my opinion, the Narcotic Anonymous (NA) model is too rigid and does not allow for appropriate opioid use. For example, the state of Washington has recently passed legislation setting an upper limit of 120mg daily, and there is now discussion of lowering that amount. I believe this is an unfortunate policy since it completely ignores the fact that each pain patient is unique. Each pain patient should be treated based on a comprehensive psychosocial evaluation, followed by specific recommendations to the prescribing referral physician.

This patient would not do well living in Washington state, since when he was referred to me he was taking 240mg of Oxycontin daily.

My initial evaluation suggested very few if any negative side effects. He was alert and clear thinking, and led an active lifestyle. He enjoyed fishing and going on walks with his dogs. He continued to drive and never had a traffic violation. He did not drink and was at peace with himself. After working with this patient, I suggested to him and his prescribing physician that he could obtain more consistent pain control if he spread out his dosing over the course of a day, and avoid a two-dose schedule, spreading it over four times a day. The patient and prescribing physician both supported this approach. After a few weeks, the patient reported more uniform pain control and his pain ratings were reduced by approximately 20%.

After gaining trust with this patient, I introduced relaxation training, augmented by biofeedback. The patient was open to this approach and reported that the relaxation techniques were helpful. His pain physician also introduced the idea of a pain infusion pump. The patient was open to the idea, but based on his previous surgical history remained somewhat doubtful. I was familiar with the pump since I consulted to Medtronic for over ten years. At that time, Medtronic was the largest manufacturer of the infusion pump. Initially, the pump was approved for cancer pain only, but in the 1990's, it received approval from the FDA for non-cancer pain.

For almost 30 years, the pain infusion pump has been used for non-cancer pain, and has generally proved to be a safe and effective option for pain management. It cannot be emphasized enough that safety depends on a rigorous selection procedure that includes a comprehensive psychosocial evaluation and a positive spinal trial. I have evaluated over 5,000 patients for implantable pain technology, both Spinal Cord Stimulators (SCS) and infusion pumps and my experience tells me it is a viable option when the patient is well selected and monitored.

Around this time, the patient's pain management physician decided to try Cymbalta. It is the first antidepressant approved for both pain and depression. It is a dual-acting medicine, blocking both the re-uptake of Serotonin and Norepinephrine. It had recently been introduced and was very expensive. The insurance carriers would not approve this medicine. The alternative was Effexor-XR (extended release), a formulation that was the precursor to Cymbalta. My own clinical experience with both preparations has been mixed. Some patients do well and benefit from these medicines, with no side effects, and others do not. Typically, this can be determined soon after initiating a trial. My patient did not do well, so it was discontinued at the 60mg level.

When I see a patient for an extended period of time, there are a number of indications that I look for to assess how a patient is doing. I look for overt behavioral indicators and at the pain rating scale, which in this case was somewhat misleading since this patient under-reported his pain. The most obvious behavior was his gait, how he carried himself. There were days when he was noticeably exhibiting pain-related behaviors, and he rarely sat down.

Another indicator is the quality of a patient's sleep. Does he report feeling rested? Is his daytime fatigue evident? With this patient, his "tells" were highly labile and varied from visit to visit. He rated his pain fairly consistently, in the 5/10 range. When you work with an under-reporter or an over-reporter, it is necessary to look for more indirect indicators of how the patient is coping with their pain.

I should also mention that this patient was an active online gambler. It did not involve a lot of money and it was certainly not a compulsive issue, but it provided hours of enjoyment that distracted him from his pain. I encourage all of my patients to pursue a hobby or activity they can do while sitting comfortably, other than watching TV. Because of their pain issues, pain patients often have a lot of down time. I recommend that they find a balance between large muscles activities and small muscle activities. Both contribute to the patient's sense of well-being and feeling that they have some control over their daily lives.

At the midpoint of our treatment time (about 7 years), he was assigned a new pain management physician at the same clinic. This caused major stress for the patient since the new physician wanted him to go off of his opioid-based medicine and try alternatives. The new suggestions included a sleep study, a trial of Lyrica, and a sleep aid (Ambien). Keep in mind that this patient was doing well, was happy with his lifestyle, and did not want to take more pills. Another suggestion was a trial of Tegretol. It did not go well. The patient complained of dizziness and nausea and his pain levels escalated. After a consultation with his new pain physician, he agreed to go back to the old regimen of 30mg of morphine four times a day and 15mg, three times a day for breakthrough pain. His pain levels went down, his mood improved, he was less antalgic and his sleep stabilized.

This experience presented a situation where the patient was succeeding with his existing treatment, but worsened with an alteration to his treatment.

The new pain physician wanted to do well by the patient but he underestimated the patient's need for maintaining what was working for him. My role during this period became more of an advocate and troubleshooter, with a heavy dose of emotional support. At this time, the plan for a trial of an intrathecal morphine pump was placed on hold. This was not a good time for the patient, and the experience undermined his confidence in his medical providers.

At this point, we shifted to a once per month schedule with an emphasis on maintenance and relapse prevention. He was medically and psychologically stable so this shift appeared reasonable. The patient continued to be active and appeared content with his quality of life. His pain levels were less labile and he continued at the same level of pain medicine with no negative side effects.

Also, at this point in treatment, the patient expressed concern over the cost of UA/drug screening since his last bill was $1,500. I reassured his pain physician that he was not drug seeking nor were there any indications that he was diverting his medicine. In my opinion, the cost of drug screening appeared to be unrealistic and onerous to the patient. Monthly screening is not medically or psychologically warranted in a patient that has a long history of stability and close monitoring from a multidisciplinary treatment model.

As I review the course of this patient's treatment, the roles of continuous monitoring, problem solving, emotional support, and advocacy were an extremely important set of behavioral tools in maintaining the patient's well-being. Not every patient is suitable for long-term maintenance therapy. There are a number of characteristics necessary to make this a worthwhile endeavor.

First, the patient must be motivated to continue this type of support. This patient confided in me that he looks forward to our monthly visits and he always feels better after each visit. For this patient, there was enough of a personal reinforcement to continue our visits, which in itself appears to be justified emotionally and financially.

Other considerations included his pain physician's encouragement to continue this adjunctive service. It is important for patients on long-term opioid pain treatment to have ongoing support since a number of issues might occur. Opioid-based treatment increases the risk of clinical depression since they are activating the central nervous system (CNS). If a pain patient is mildly depressed, and most are, adding a CNS opioid-depressing influence can compound the depression, so that it becomes more of a clinical issue. Physicians in general do not have the time or skill to identify and treat clinical depression, so it is prudent for a pain to be involved in long-term monitoring and support.

In the past few years, this patient has done well, remaining active, enjoying his hobbies, and leading a full life. His wife has not called me with instructions for several years and I know if something was amiss she would let me know!

Notes

Chapter 1 – A History of Pain

1. Damasio, AR. (1994) *Descartes' Error*. New York: Putnam.
2. Decartes, R.(1664) *Traite de l'Homme*, Paris: Angot, 1664.
3. Haldane, ES. (1968) *The Philosophical Works of Descartes*. Cambridge: Cambridge University Press. (original work written 1628).
4. Head, H. (1920) *Studies in Neurology, Vol. 2*, Oxford: Oxford University Press.
5. Livingston, WK. (1998) *Pain and Suffering*. Seattle, WA: IASP Press.
6. Livingston, WK. (1943) *Pain Mechanisms: A Physiologic Interpretation of Causalogia and Its Related States*. New York: MacMillian Co.
7. Melzack R, Casey KL. (1968) *Sensory, Motivational and Central Control Determinants of Pain: A New Conceptual Model*. In D. Kenshalo (Ed.), The Skin Senses, pp 423–443. Springfield, IL.: Charles C. Thomas.
8. Melzack R, Wall PD. (1965) *Pain Mechanisms: A New Theory, Science*, 150, pp 971–979.
9. Melzack R, Wall PD. (1988) *The Challenge of Pain*. New York: Penguin Books.
10. Rey, R. (1993) *History of Pain*, Paris: La Decounette.
11. Sherrington, CS. (1906) *The Integrative Action of the Nervous System*. New York: Charles Scribner's Sons.

<u>Note</u>: All of the major contributors covered in this chapter are available online. For more information about the history of pain, it is recommended that you visit The John Liebskind History of Pain Collection at the Louise M. Darling Biomedical Library at UCLA.

Chapter 2 – The Nature of Pain

1. Basbaum, AF, Fields HL. (1978) Endogenous pain control mechanisms: Review and hypothesis. *Ann Neurol. (4)* 451–62.
2. Bonica, JJ. (1980) *Pain*. New York: Raven.
3. Casey, KL, Bushnell MC. (2000) *Pain Imaging*. Seattle, WA: IASP Press.
4. Fields, HL. (1987) *Pain*. New York: McGraw-Hill.
5. Head, HH. (1911)Sensory disturbances from sensory cerebral lesions. *Brain (34)* 102–254.
6. Julien, N, Arenault, P., Marchand, S. (2005) Widespread pain in fibromyalgia is associated to a deficit of endogenous pain inhibition. *Pain (114)* 295–302.
7. Le Bars, O. (2002)The whole body receptive field of dorsal horn multireceptive neurons. *Brain Research Rev (40)* 29–44.
8. Livingston, WK. (1998)*Pain and Suffering*. Seattle, WA: IASP Press.
9. Loeser, JD, Ford, WE. (1983) Chronic Pain, In: Carr, JE., Dengerink, HA. (Eds.) Behavioral

science in the practice of medicine. New York: Elsevier Biomedical; 1983. P. 331–45.

10. Marchand, S. (2012) *The phenomenon of pain*. Seattle, WA: IASP Press.

11. Melzack, R, Wall, PD. (1965) Pain mechanisms: a new theory. *Sci Am (150)* 971–9.

12. Olson, KA., Bedder MD, et al. (1997) Psychological variables associated with outcome in spinal cord stimulation trials. *Neuromodulation (1)* 6–13.

13. Olson, KA. (1997) Prognostic value of psychological testing in patients undergoing spinal cord stimulation. *Pain Medicine Journal (3)* 31–33.

14. Olson, KA. (1996) The value of multiple sources of data in decision making. *Pain Forum (5)* 104–106.

15. Olson, KA. (2011) Identifying psychological factors that influence surgical outcomes. *Practical Pain Management, September* 111–116.

16. Russell, IJ. (1998) Neurochemical pathogenesis of fibromyalgia. *Z Rheumatol (57)* 63–66.

17. Treede, RD., Apkarian, AV., Bromm, B., Greenspan, JD., Lenz, FA. (2000) Cortical representation of pain: Functional characterization of nociceptive areas near the lateral sulcus. *Pain (87)* 113–119.

18. Willis, WD. (1985) Nociceptive pathways anatomy and physiology of nociceptive ascending pathways. *Philos Trans R Soc Lond B Biol Sci 1985 (308)* 253–70.

Chapter 3 – Pain Assessment

1. Bergner, M., Bobbitt, RA., Carter, WB., Gibson, BS. (1981) The Sickness Impact Profile: Development and final revision of a health status measure. *Medical Care, 19,* 787–805. Boden, SD., Davis, DO., Dina, TS., Pattonas, NJ., Wiesel, SW. (1990) Abnormal magnetic resonance scans of the lumbar spine in asymptomatic subjects. *Journal of Bone and Joint Surgery. 72A.*403–408.

2. DeGood, DE. Shutty, MS. (1992) Assessment of pain beliefs, coping and self-efficacy. I DC Turk and Melzack (Eds) *Handbook of Pain Assessment* (pp 214–234). New York: Guilford Press.

3. Deyo, RA. (1986)The early diagnostic evaluation of patients with low back pain. *Journal of General Internal Medicine. I,* 328–338.

4. Dworkin, RH., Turk, DC., Wyrwick, KW. (2008) Interpreting the clinical importance of treatment outcomes in chronic pain clinical trials: IMMPACT recommendations. *Journal of Pain, 9,* 105–121.

5. Flor, H., Turk, DC. (1989) Psychophysiology of Chronic Pain: Do chronic pain patients exhibit symptom-specific psychophysiological responses? *Psychological Bulletin, 105,* 215–259.

6. Fordyce, WE. (1976) *Behavioral Methods for Chronic Pain and Illness*. St. Louis, MO: Mosby.

7. Freedman, R. Ianni, P. Wenig, P. (1983) Behavioral Treatment of Raynaud's Disease. *Journal of Consulting and Clinical Psychology, 51,* 539–549.

8. Hing, E., Cherry, DK., Woodwell, DA.(2004) National Ambulatory Medical Care Survey: 2004 Summary Hyattsville, MD.

9. Jensen, MC., Brandt-Zawadski, MN., Obuchowski, N., Modic, MT., Malkasian Ross, JS. (1994) Magnetic Resonance Imaging of the lumbar spine in people with pack pain. *New England Journal of Medicine, 331*, 69–73.

10. Jensen, MP., Karoly, P., Hunger, R. (1987) The development and preliminary validation of an instrument to assess patients' attitudes toward pain. *Journal of Psychosomatic Research, 31*, 393–400. 1987.

11. Kerns, RD., Turk, DC., Rudy, TE. (1985) The West Haven-Yale Multdimensional Pain Inventory (WHYMPI). *Pain, 23*, 345–356.

12. Lazarus, RS., Folkman, S. (1984) *Stress Appraisal and Coping.* New York: Springer.

13. Lethbridge-Cejku, M., Vickerie, J. (2005) Summary of health statistics for US adults: National Health-Interview Survey, National Center for Health Statistics.

14. Melzack, R. (1975) The McGill Pain Questionnaire: Major properties and scoring methods. *Pain, 13*, 277–299.

15. Melzack, R., Casey, KL. (1968) Sensory, Motivational and Central Control Determinants of Pain: A New Conceptual Model. In D Kenshalo (Editor). *The Skin Senses,* pp 423–443. Springfield, IL: Thomas.

16. Melzack, R., Torgerson, WS. (1971) On the Language of Pain. *Anesthesiology, 34*, 50–59.

17. National Center for Health Statistics (NCHS). Health, United States, with chart book on trends in the health of Americans. Hyattsville, MD. 2006.

18. NIH Technology Assessment Panel on Integration of Behavioral and Relaxation Approaches into the Treatment of Chronic Pain and Insomnia. *Journal of Medical Association, 276*, 313–318. 1996.

19. Olson, KA. (2011) *Handbook of Pain Assessment, Third Edition,* Editors Turk D Melzack R. (Book Review) *Practical Pain Management. July/August. 2011.*

20. Olson, KA. (2011) Pain and sleep: a delicate balance, (exclusive report) *Practical Pain Management. Nov/Dec. 2011.*

21. Rosenatiel, AK., Keefe, FJ. (1983) The Use of Coping Strategies in Chronic Low Back Pain Patients: Relationship to Patient Characteristics and Current Adjustment. *Pain, 17*, 33–44.

22. Stone, A., Broderick, J., Shiffman, S., Schwartz, JE. (2004)Understanding Recall of Weekly Pain From a Momentary Assessment Perspective: Absolute Agreement, Between and Withing Person Consistence and Judged Change in Weekly Pain. *Pain, 107*, 61–69.

23. Sullivan, MJL., Stanish, W., Waite, H. (1998) Catastrophizing, pain and disability in patients with soft-tissue injuries. *Pain 77*, 253–260.

24. Thieme K Turk D. (2006) Heterogeneity of psychophysiological stress responses in fibromyalgia syndrome. *Arthritis Research and Therapy, 8* (1), R9.

25. Turk D., Melzack R., (Eds.) (2011) *Handbook of Pain Assessment.* New York: The Guilford Press.

26. Turk, D., Rudy, TE. (1990) Neglected factors in chronic pain treatment outcome studies: referral patterns, failure to enter treatment and attrition. *Pain. 43*, 7–26.

27. Skinner, B.F. (1965) *Science and Human Behavior.* New York: Free Press.

Chapter 4 – The Treatment of Pain

1. Beaulieu, P., Lussier, D., Porreca, F., Dickenson, AH. (edts.) (2010) *Pharmacology of Pain.* Seattle, WA: IASP Press.

2. Beck, AT., Rush, AJ., Shaw, BF., Emery, G. (1979) *Cognitive Therapy of Depression*, New York: Guilford Press.

3. Benson, H. (1969)*The Relaxation Response,* New York: Harper.

4. Black, AR., Gatchel, RJ., Deredorff, WW., Guyer, RD. (2003) *The Psychology of Spine Surgery*, Washington DC: American Psychological Association.

5. Cameron, T. (2004) Safety and efficacy of spinal cord stimulation for the treatment of chronic pain: a 20-year literature review. *J Neurosurgery, 100 (3 Suppl Spine)*: 254–267.

6. Caudill, MA. (2009) *Managing Pain Before It Manages You*, Third Edition, New York: Guilford Press,.

7. Chou, E., Fanciullo, GJ., Fine, PG. (2009) Clinical guidelines for the use of chronic opioid therapy in chronic non-cancer pain. *The Journal of Pain,10*(2):113–130.

8. Compass, BE., Haaga, DAF., Keefe, FJ., Leitenbery H., Williams, DA. (1998) A Sampling of empirically supported psychological treatments from health psychology: smoking, chronic pain, cancer and bulimia nervosa. *J Consult Clin Psychol., 66*:89–112.

9. Deer, TR., Prager, J., Levy, R,. et al. (2012)Polyanalgesic consensus conference 2012: recommendations for the management of pain by intrathecal (intraspinal) drug delivery: report of an interdisciplinary expert panel. *Neuromodulation, 15(5)*:436–464.

10. Deyo, RA., Walsh, NE., et al. (1990)A controlled trial of transcutaneous electrical nerve stimulation (TENS) and exercise for chronic low back pain. *N Engl J Med. 322*:1627-34.

11. Fishman, SM. (2012) *Responsible Opioid Prescribing, Second Edition*, Washington DC: Waterford Life Sciences.

12. Flor, H., Nikolajsen, L., Jensen, ST. (2006) Phantom limb pain: a case of maladaptive CNS plasticity? *Nat Rev Neurosci, 7*:873-81.

13. Ghia, JN., Mao, W., Toomey, TC., Gregg, JM. (1976) Acupuncture and chronic pain mechanisms. *Pain, 2*:285-99.

14. Jacobson, E. (1938) *Progressive Relaxation.* Chicago, IL: University of Chicago Press.

15. Jensen MP. (2011) *Hypnosis for Chronic Pain Management.* New York: Oxford University Press.

16. Keefe, FJ., LeFebvre, J. (1994) Pain Behavior Concepts: Controversies, Current Status, and Future Directions. In: Gebhart, G., Hammond, DL., Jenson, TS., (Eds.) *Proceedings of the 7th World Congress on Pain, Progress in Pain Research and Management, Vol. 2.* Seattle, WA: IASP Press. Pp 127–147.

17. Leonard, G., Cloutier, C., Marchand, S. (2011)Reduced analgesic effect of acupuncture-like TENS but not conventional TENS in opioid-treated patients. *J Pain. 12*-213-21.

18. Lewinsohn, PM., et al. (1986) *Control Your Depression.* Englewood Cliffs, NJ: Prentice-Hall.

19. Lipman, AG., Jackson, KC II. *Opioid Pharmaco Therapy.* In Warfield CA, Bajwa ZH, (Eds.)

Principles and practice of Pain Medicine, New York: McGraw-Hill. pp 139–147.

20. Luthe, W. (1969) *Autogenic Therapy.* New York, Grune and Stratton.

21. Marchand, S. (2012)*The Phenomenon of Pain,* Seattle, WA: IASP Press

22. Marchand, S., Charest, J., et al. (1993) Is TENS purely a placebo effect? A controlled study on chronic low back pain. *Pain, 54*:99-106.

23. Marchand, S., Li, J., Charest, J. (1995) Effects of caffeine on analgesia from transcutaneous electrical nerve stimulation. *N Engl J Med., 333*:325-6.

24. Melzack, R. (1990) The Tragedy of Needless Pain, *Sci Am, 262*:27-33.

25. Melzack, R., Stillwell, DM., Fox, EJ. (1977) Trigger points and acupuncture points for pain: Correlations and implications. *Pain, 3*:3-23.

26. Miller, EE., Halpern, S. *Letting Go of Stress.* www.DrMiller. com and www.innerpeacemusic. com

27. Moore, SR., Shurman, J. (1997) Combined neuromuscular electrical stimulation and transcutaneous electrical nerve stimulation for treatment of chronic back pain: A double-blind, repeated measures comparison. *Arch Phys Med Rehabil., 78*:55-60.

28. North, RB., Kidd, DH., Farrokhl, F., Plantadosi, SA. (2005) Spinal cord stimulation versus repeated lumbosacral spine surgery for chronic pain: A randomized controlled trial. *Neurosurgery, 56(1)*:98-106.

29. Oaklander, AL., North, RB. (2001) Failed Back Surgery Syndrome. In: Loser J, Butler SH, Chapman CR, Turk DC (Eds). *Bonica's Management of Pain, Third Edition.* Philadelphia: Lippincott, Williams and Wilkins, pp 1540–1549.

30. Oakley, J., Prager, J. (2002) Spinal cord stimulation: Mechanisms of action. *Spine. 2002;27(22)*:2574-2583.

31. Park, A., Suddath, C., Cloud, J. (2011) Chronic pain, *Time mag.* Pp 63–88, March 7, 2011.

32. Shor, RE., Orne, EC. (1962) *Harvard Group Scale of Hypnotic Susceptibility, Form A,* Palo Alto, CA: Consulting Psychologist Press.

33. Simmons, DG. (2008) New views of myofascial trigger points: Etiology and diagnosis. *Arch Phys Med Rehabil., 89*:157-9.

34. Travell, J., Simmons, D. (1983) *Myofascial Pain and Dysfunction: The Trigger Point Manual.* New York: Williams and Wilkins.

35. Tellegan A, Alkinson G. (1974) Openness to Absorbing and self-altering experiences (Absorption) as related to hypnotic susceptibility. *J of Abnormal Psychology. Vol 83 (3)* 268–277.

36. Turk, DC. (1997) Psychological aspects of pain In: *Expert Pain Management.* Springhouse, PA: Springhouse Corp.

37. Webster, LR., et al. (2010) Select Medical-Legal Reviews of Unintentional Overdose Deaths. Presented at the 26th Annual Meeting of AAPM, February 3–6, 2010. San Antonio, TX.

38. World Health Organization: Ensuring Balance in National Policies on Controlled Substance 2011. http://www.painpolicy.wisc.edu/publict/IIWHOGLS/WHOGLS.pdf

Chapter 5 – Pain and Sleep

1. Baghdoyan, HA. (2006) Hyperalgesia induced by REM sleep loss: A phenomenon in search of a mechanism. *Sleep, (29)* 137–139.
2. Baker FC., Driver, HS., Paiker, J., et al. (2002) Acetaminophen does not affect 24 hour body temperature or sleep in the luteal phase of the menstrual cycle. *J Appl Physiol, (92)* 1684–1691.
3. Boardman HF., Thomas, E., Millson, DS., Croft, PR. (2006) The natural history of headache: Predictors of onset and recovery. *Cephalagia, (26)* 1080–1088.
4. Cairns, BE. (2007) Pain medication and sleep quality. In: *Sleep and Pain.* Levigne G, et al. Seattle, WA: IASP Press.
5. Carskadon, MA., Dement, WC. (2005) Normal Human Sleep: An Overview. In: Kryger, MH., Roth, T., Dement, WC. (Eds.). *Principles and Practices of Sleep Medicine, Vol 4.* Philadelphia PA: Elsevier Sanders, pp13–23.
6. Choiniere M., Racine M., Raymond-Shaw, I. (2007) Epidemiology of pain and sleep disturbances and their reciprocal interrelationships. In: Levigne, G., et al. *Sleep and Pain.* Seattle, WA: IASP Press.
7. Colombo, B., Annovazzi, POL., Comi, G. (2006) Mechanisms and treatment of neuropathic pain. *Neural Sci. (27)* 5183–5189.
8. Damasio, A. (2010) Self Comes to Mind. NY, NY: Vintage Books.
9. Doghramji, K. (2007) Melatonin and its receptors: A new class of sleep-promoting agents. *JCSM (Supplement)(3)* 517–523.
10. Erman M., Seiden D., Zamint G., Sainati S., Zhang J. (2006) An efficacy, safety, and dose response study of Ramelton in patients with chronic primary insomnia. *Sleep Med. (7)* 17–24.
11. Finan ,PH,. Goodin, BR., Smith, MT. (2013)The Association of Sleep and Pain: An Update and a Path Forward. *Jour. Of Pain. (14)* 1539–1552.
12. Hamet, P., Tromblay, J. (2006) Genetics of sleep-wake cycle and its disorders. *Metabolism (55)* 57–512
13. Hauri, P., Linde, S. (1996) *No More Sleepless Nights.* NY, NY. John Wiley & Sons, Inc.;
14. Haythornthwaite, JA., Heget, Kerns, RD. (1991) Development of a sleep diary for chronic pain patients. *J Pain Symptom Manag. (6)* 65–72.
15. Hindmarch, I., Dawson. J., Stanley, N. (2005) A double blind study in healthy volunteers to assess the effects on sleep of pregablin compared with alprazolam and placebo. *Sleep* 2005; *(28)* 187–193.
16. Jensen, M., Turk, D. (2014)Contributions of psychology to the understanding and treatment of people with chronic pain. *Am. Psychologist, (2)* 105–118.
17. Johns, MW. (1991)A new method for measuring daytime sleepiness: The Epworth Sleepiness Scale. *Sleep (6)* 540–545.
18. Karim, A., Tolbert, D., Cao, C. (2006) Disposition kinetics and tolerance of escalating single doses of ramelton a high-affinity MTI and MTZ melatonin receptor agonist indicated for

the treatment of insomnia. *J Clin Pharmacol (46)* 140–148.

19. Lavie, P. (1997) Melatonin: role in gating nocturnal rise in sleep propensity. J *Biol Rhythms, (12)* 657–665.

20. Lavie, P., Hahir, M., Lorder, M., et al. (1991)Nonsteroidal anti-inflammatory drug therapy in rheumatoid arthritis. Lack of association between clinical improvement and effects on sleep. *Arthritis Rheum. (34)* 655–659.

21. Lydic, R., Baghdayan, HA. (2005) Sleep anesthesiology and the neurobiology of arousal state control. *Anesthesiology (103)* 779–787.

22. Lyngberg, AC., Rasmussen, BK., Jorgensen, T., Jensen, R. (2005) Has the prevalence of migraine and tension-type headache changed over a 12 year period? A Danish population survey. *Eur J Epidemiol, (20)* 243-249.

23. Migot, E., Taheri, S., Nishino, S. (2002) Sleeping with the hypothalamus: Emerging therapeutic targets for sleep disorders. *Nat Neurosci. (5)* 1071-1075.

24. Morin, CM., Kowatch, RA., Wade, KB. (1989) Behavioral management of sleep disturbances secondary to chronic pain. *J Behav Ther Exp Psychiatry (20)* 295-302.

25. Mork, PJ., Nilsen, TI. (2012) Sleep problems and risk of fibromyalgia: Longitudinal data on an adult female population in Norway. *Arthritis Rheum. (64)* 281-284.

26. Neubauer,D. (2007) The evolution and development of insomnia pharmacotherapies. *JCSM (3)* 311-315.

27. Odegard, SS., Sand ,T., Engstrom, M., Stovner, LJ., Zwart, JA., Hagen, K. (2011) The long-term effect of insomnia on primary headaches: A prospective population-based cohort study (HUNT- 2 and HUNT -3) *Headache, (51)* 570-580.

28. Olson, KA. (2011) Pain and sleep: A delicate balance. *Pract Pain Manage. 11 (9)* 46-47.

29. Olson, KA. (2013) The nature of pain. *Pract Pain Manage. October 2013;* 31-40

30. Roehrs, T., Hyde, M., Blaisdell, B., Greenwald, M., Roth, T. (2006) Sleep loss and REM sleep loss are hyperalgesic. *Sleep, (29)* 145-151.

31. Saarto, T., Wiffen, P. (2005) Antidepressants for neuropathic pain. *Cochrane Database Syst Rev.* CD005454

32. Saper, CB., Scammell, TB., Lu, J. (2005) Hypothalamic regulation of sleep and circadian rhythms. *Nature, (437)* 1257-1263.

33. Sharpley, AL., Williamson, DJ., Attenburrow, ME., et al. (1996) The effects of paroxetine and netazodone on sleep: A placebo controlled trial. *Psycho Pharmacology (BERL) (126)* 50-54.

34. Smith, MT., Haythornthwaite, JA. (2004) How do sleep disturbances and chronic pain inter-relate? Insights from the longitudinal and cognitive-behavioral clinical trials literature. *Sleep Med Rev. (8)* 119-132.

35. Smith, MT., et al. (2000) Sleep quality and pre-sleep arousal in chronic pain. *J Behav Med. (23)* 1-13.

36. Staner, L., Kerkhots, M., Detroux, D., et al. (1995) Acute subchronic and withdrawal sleep EEG changes during treatment with paroxetine and amitriptyline: A double-blind randomized trial in major depression. *Sleep.* 1995; (18) 470-477.

37. Wisor, JP., Nishino, S., Sora, I., et al. (2001)Dopaminergic role in stimulant-induced wakefulness. *J Neurosci., (21)* 1787-1794.

38. Zadra, A., Manzini, C. (2007) Pain in dreams and nightmares in sleep and pain. In: *Sleep and Pain.* Levigne, G., et al., Seattle, WA: IASP Press.

Chapter 6 – Age and Pain

1. American Geriatrics Society Panel on the Pharmacological Management of Persistent Pain in Older Persons. *Pain Medicine.* 2009. (10): 1062-1083.

2. American Pain Society Task Force on Pediatric Chronic Pain Management. (2012) Assessment and Management of Children with Chronic Pain: A position statement from the American Pain Society. Retrieved from http://www.americanpainsociety.org/uploads/pdfs/aps12-pcp.pdf

3. Anand, KJ., Phil, D., Craig, KD. (1996) New perspectives on the definition of pain. *Pain. (67):* 3-6.

4. Anand, KJ, Phil, D., Hickey, PR. (1987) Pain and its effect in the human neonate and fetus. *N Engl J Med.* 1987. (317): 1321-29.

5. Anand, KJ, Scalzo, FM. (2000) Can adverse neonatal experiences alter brain development and subsequent behavior? *Biol Neonate.* (77): 69-82.

6. Benedetti, F., Arduino, C., Vighetti, S., Asteggiano, G., Tarenzi, L., & Rainero, I. (2004). Pain reactivity in Alzheimer patients with different degrees of cognitive impairment and brain electrical activity deterioration. *Pain, 111*(1-2), 22-29.http://dx.doi.org/10.1016/j.pain.2004.05.015

7. Beyer, JE., et al. (1990) Discordance between self-report and behavioral pain measures in children aged 3-7 years after surgery. J *Pain Symptom Mang. (5)*: 350-56.

8. Campo, JV., et al. (2007) Physical and emotional health of mother's of youth with functional abdominal pain. *Arch of Ped and Adolescent Med. (2)*: 131-137.

9. Cannon, KT., et al. (2006) Potentially inappropriate medication use in elderly patients receiving home health care: A retrospective data analysis. *Am Jour of Geriatric Pharm. (4):* 134-143.

10. Centers for Disease Control and Prevention. (2013). *The State of Aging and Health in America 2013.* Atlanta, GA.

11. Chen, Q, et al. (2011) Characteristics of persistent pain associated with sleep difficulty in older adults: The maintenance of balance, independent living, intellect and rest in the elderly (MOBILIZE) Boston Study, Jour of the *Am Geriatrics Society, (59)*: 1385-1392.

12. Chou, KL. (2007) Reciprocal relationship between pain and depression in older adults: Evidence from the English Longitudinal Study of Aging. *Jour of Affective Disorders. (102)*: 115-123.

13. Claar, RL, et al. (2008) Parental response to children's pain: The moderating impact of children's emotional distress on symptoms and disability. *Pain, (1)*: 172-179.

14. Cohen, L., et al. (2010) Parenting an adolescent with chronic pain: An investigation of how

a taxonomy of adolescent functioning relates to parent distress. *J of Ped Psych., (7):* 748-757.

15. Corbett, A., et al. (2012)Assessment and treatment of pain in people with dementia. *Nature Reviews Neurology, (5):* 264-274.

16. Corran, TM. (1997) The classification of patients with persistent pain: Age as a contributing factor. *The Clinical J of Pain, (13):* 207-214.

17. Denard, PJ., et al. (2010) Back pain neurogenic symptoms and physical function in relation to spondylothesis among elderly men. *The Spine Journal, (10):* 865-873.

18. Gleicher, Y., et al. (2011)A prospective study of mental health care for comorbid depressed mood in older adults with painful osteoarthritis. *BMC Psychiatry, (11):* 147-157.

19. Hechler, T., et al. (2011)Parental catastrophizing about their child's chronic pain: Are mothers and fathers different? *European J of Pain, (5):* 515.el-.eq.

20. Huguet, A., Mira J. (2008) The severity of chronic pediatric pain: An epidemiological study. *The J of Pain (9):* 226-236.

21. Huxholt, O., et al. (2013)The dynamic interplay of social network characteristics, subjective well-being and health: The costs and benefits of socio-emotional selectivity theory. *Psychology and Aging, (28):* 3-16.

22. Jensen, MP., et al. (2011) Psychosocial factors and adjustment to persistent pain in persons with physical disabilities: A systematic review. *Arch of Physical Med and Rehab., (92):* 146-160.

23. Kemper, KJ., et al. (2000) On pins and needles? Pediatric pain patients experience with acupuncture. *Pediatrics, (105):* 941-47.

24. Langley, PC. (2011) The prevalence correlates and treatment of pain in the European Union. *Current Medical Research and Opinion, (27):* 463-480.

25. Lavigene, JV. (1986) Psychological aspects of painful medical conditions in children: Personality factors, family characteristics and treatment. *Pain, (27):* 147-69.

26. Marchand, S. (2012)*The Phenomenon of Pain.* Seattle WA: IASP Press.

27. McAuliffe, L., et al. (2009)Pain assessment in older people with dementia: Literature review. *Jour of Adv Nursing, (1):* 2-10.

28. McCarthy, LH., et al. (2009) Persistent pain and obesity in elderly people: Results from the Einstein Aging Study. *J of the Am Geriatrics Society, (57):* 115-119.

29. McGrath, PA.(1990) Pain in children. New York: Guilford. p 466.

30. McGraw, MB. (1941)Neural maturation as exemplified in the changing reactions of the infant to pin prick. *Child Dev., (12):* 31-42.

31. Miller, SW. Therapeutic drug monitoring in the geriatric patient. In JE Murphy (Ed) *American Society of Health Systems Pharmacists* (4th Ed, pp 45-71).

32. Olson, KA. (2014)Pain and sleep: Understanding the interrelationship. *Practical Pain Management, (14):* 59-65.

33. Palermo, TM. (2012) *Cognitive-Behavioral Therapy for Chronic Pain in Children and Adolescents.* NY: Oxford University Press.

34. Perquin, CW., et al. (2000) Pain in children and adolescents: A common experience. *Pain, 87* (1):51-58.

35. Puchalski, M., Hummel, P. (2002) The reality of neonatal pain. *Adv Neonatal Pain. Adv Neonatal Care, (2):* 233-44.

36. Rhee, H. (2003)Physical symptoms in children and adolescents. *An Rev of Nursing Research. (21):* 95-121.

37. Rolita, L., Freeman, M. (2008) Over-the-counter medication use in older adults. *Jour of Gerontological Nursing, (34):* 8-17.

38. Routledge, PA, et al. (2004) Adverse drug reactions in elderly patients. *British Jour of Clinical Pharm., (57):* 121-126.

39. Schechter, NL, et al. (2009) In SM Fishman, et al (Eds) *Bonica's Management of Pain* (4th Ed). pp 767-782. Philadelphia, PA: Lippincott Williams and Wilkins

40. Strine, TW., et al. (2005) Health related quality of life health risk behaviors and disability among adults with pain related activity difficulty. *Am J of Geriatric Psychiatry. (95):* 2042-2048.

41. Swafford, LI., Allan, D. (1968) Pain relief in pediatric patient. *Med Clin North Am., (52):* 131-137.

42. Szczerbinska, KK., et al. (2012) Depressive symptoms decline and under treatment increases with age in home care and institutional settings. *The Am Jour of Geriatric Psychiatry, (20):* 1045-1056.

43. Trautmann, E., et al. (2006) (Psychological treatment of recurrent headache in children and adolescents: A meta analysis. *Cephalgia (12):* 1411-1426.

44. Tsang, A, et al. (2008) Common persistent pain conditions in developed and developing countries: Gender and age differences and comorbidity with depression anxiety disorders. *The J of Pain (9):* 883-891.

45. US Census Bureau (2011 November). The older population : 2010. Retrieved from http://www.census.gov/prod/cen2010/briefs/c2010bro9.pdf.

46. Valentine, RJ., et al. (2011) The association of adiposity, physical activity and inflammation with fatigue in older adults. *Brain, Behavior and Immunity, (25):* 1482-1490.

47. Verdu' E, et al. (2000) Influence of aging on peripheral nerve function and regeneration. *Jour of the Peripher Nervous System, (5):* 191-208.

48. Williamson, GM. (2000) Extending the activity restriction model of depressed affect: Evidence from a sample of breast cancer patients. *Health Psychology, (19):* 339-347.

49. Wolf N, et al. (2010) Determinants of somatic complaints in 18 month old children: The generation R study. *J of Ped Psych., (3):* 306-316.

50. Wooten JM. Pharmeotherapy considerations in elderly adults. (2012) *Southern Med Jour., (105):* 437-445.

Chapter 7 – Gender and Pain

1. Aloisi, AM., et al. (2005) Gender-related effects of chronic non-malignant pain and opioid therapy on plasma levels of macrophage migration inhibitory factor (MIF) *Pain, 115:* 142-51.

2. Aloisi, AM., Monifazi, M. (2006) Sex hormones, central nervous system and pain. *Horm Behv., 50*:1-7.

3. Anderson, GB. (1999) Epidemiological features of chronic low-back pain. *Lancet 354:* 581-5.

4. Banks, SM., Kerns, RD. (1996) Explaining high rates of depression in chronic pain: a diathesis-stress framework. *Psychol Bull, 119*: 95-110.

5. Bolton, JE. (1994) Psychological distress and disability in back pain patients evidence of sex differences. *J Psychosomatic Res, 38*: 849-58.

6. Bruehl, S., et al. (2002) The relationship between resting blood pressure and acute pain sensitivity in healthy normotensives and chronic back sufferers: the effects of opioid blockage. *Pain; 100*: 191-201.

7. Carroll, LJ., et al. (2004) Depression as a risk factor for onset of an episode of troublesome neck and low back pain. *Pain, 107*: 134-9.

8. Cousins, N. (1979) *Anatomy of an Illness.* Norton & Co. NY.

9. Craft, RM. (2003) Sex differences in opioid analgesia: "from mouse to man". Clin J *Pain, 19*: 175-86.

10. Cutolo, M., Accardo, S. (1991) Sex hormones, HLA and rheumatoid arthritis. *Clin Exp Rheumatol, 9*: 641-6.

11. Dao, TT., LeResche, L. (2000) Gender differences in pain. J Orofac *Pain, 14*: 169-84.

12. Edwards, RR., et al. (2004) Catastrophizing as a mediator of sex differences pain: differential defects for daily pain versus laboratory induced pain. *Pain, 111*: 571-77.

13. Edwards, RR., et al. (2000) Sex-specific effects of pain related anxiety on adjustment to chronic pain. *Clin J Pain, 16*: 46-53.

14. Fearon, I., et al. (1996) "Booboos": the study of everyday pain among young children. *Pain, 68*: 55-62.

15. Fillingin, RB., Maixner W. (1995) Gender differences in the responses to noxious stimuli. *Pain Forum, 4:* 209-21.

16. Fillingin, RB. (2000) *Sex, Gender and Pain.* Progress in pain research and management, vol 17. Seattle, WA: IASP Press

17. Fillingin, RB., et al. (2002) Sex differences in perceptual and cardiovascular responses to pain: The influence of a perceived ability manipulation. *J of Pain, 3*: 439-445.

18. Frot, M., et al. (2004) Sex differences in pain perception and anxiety. A psychophysical study with topical capsaicin. *Pain, 108*: 230-6.

19. Gaumond, I., et al. (2005) Specificity of female and male sex hormones on excitatory and inhibitory phases of formalin-induced nociceptive responses. *Brain Res, 1052*: 105-11.

20. Goffaux P, et al. (2011) Sex differences in perceived pain are affected by an anxious brain. *Pain, 52*: 2065-73.

21. Haley WE, et al. (1985) Depression in chronic pain patients relation to pain, activity and sex differences. *Pain, 23*: 337-43.

22. Haywood, SA., et al. (1999) Fluctuating estrogen and progesterone receptor expression in brainstem norepinephrine neurons through the RAT estrous cycle. *Endocrinology, 140*: 355-63.

23. Keefe, FJ., et al. (2004) Gender differences in pain coping, mood and individuals having osteo-arthritic knee pain: a within-day analysis. *Pain* 110: 571-77.

24. Kuba, T., Quinones-Jenab, V. (2005) The role of female gonadal hormones in behavioral sex differences in persistent and chronic pain: clinical versus preclinical studies. *Brain Research Bulletin 66*: 179-88.

25. Marchand, S. (2012) *The Phenomenon of Pain*. Seattle, WA: IASP Press.

26. Meana, M. (1998)The meeting of pain and depression: co-morbidity in women. *Can J Psychiatry 43*: 893-9.

27. Mechanic, D. (1964)The influence of mothers on their children's health attitudes and behavior. *Pediatrics, 33*: 444-53.

28. Meiri, H. (2000) Is synaptic transmission modulated by progesterone? *Brain Res, 385:* 196-6.

29. Miaskowski C, et al. (2000) Sex related differences in analgesic responses. In: Fillingin RB, ed. *Sex, Gender and Pain*. Seattle, WA: IASP Press; 209-30.

30. Willer, JC, et al. (1981) Stress-induced analgesia in humans: endogenous opioids and naloxone-reversible depression of pain reflexes. *Science, 212*: 689-91.

31. Rhudy, JL., Meagher, MW. (2000) Fear and anxiety: divergent effects on human pain thresholds. *Pain, 84*: 65-75.

32. Rhudy, JL, Williams AE. (2005) Gender differences in pain: do emotions play a role? *Gend Med, 2*: 208-26.

33. Riley, JL, et al. (1998) Sex differences in the perception of noxious experimental stimuli: a meta-analysis. *Pain, 74*: 181-7.

34. Riley, JL, et al. (2001) Sex differences in negative emotional responses to chronic pain. *J Pain, 2*: 354-9.

35. Robinson, ME, Riley, JL. (1999) The role of emotion in pain. In: Gatchel RJ, Turk, DC. Eds. *Psychosocial Factors in Pain*, 1st ed. NY: Guilford Press. P 74-88.

36. Robinson, JE., Short, RV. (1977) Changes in breast sensitivity in puberty during the menstrual cycle and at parturition. *Br Med J, 1:* 1188-91.

37. Rovensky, J., et al. (2005) Hormone concentrations in synovial fluid of patients with rheumatoid arthritis. *Clin Exp Rheumatol, 23*: 292-6.

38. Sarlani, E., et al. (2004) Sex differences in temporal summation of pain and after sensations following repetitive noxious mechanical stimulation. *Pain, 109*: 115-123.

39. Tang. J., Gibson SJ. (2005) A psychophysical evaluation of the relationship between trait anxiety, pain perception and induced state anxiety. *J Pain, 6:* 612-9.

40. Tremblay, LG., et al. (2014) Sex differences in the neural representation of pain unpleasantness. *J of Pain,15:* 867-77.

41. Wallbott, HG., Scherer, KR. (1991) Stress specificities: differential effects of coping style, gender and type of stressors on autonomic arousal, facial expression and subjective feeling. *J Pers Soc Psychol, 61*: 147-56.

42. Zubieta, JK., et al. (1999) Gender and age influences on human brain mu – opioid receptor binding measured by PET. *Am J, 156*: 842-8.

Chapter 8 – Pain and Surgery

1. Burchiel, K.J, Olson, KA., et al. (1996) Prognostic factors of spinal cord stimulation for chronic back and leg pain. *Neurosurgery, Vol. 36, No. 6*, pp. 1101-1111.
2. Olson, KA. (1997) Prognostic Value of Psychological Testing in Patients Undergoing Spinal Cord Stimulation. *Pain Medicine Journal, Vol. 3, No. 1*, pp. 31-33, (commentary).
3. Olson, KA. & Bedder, MD., et al. (1997) Psychological Variables Associated with Outcome in Spinal Cord Stimulation Trials. *Neuromodulation, Vol. 1, No. 1*, pp. 6-13.

Chapter 9 – Motivation and Trust

1. Benson, H. (1975) *The Relaxation Response.* New York, NY; Harper.
2. Caudill, MA. (2009) *Managing Pain Before it Manages You.* New York, NY: Guilford Press.
3. Luthe, Wolfgang, Schultz, JH. (1969)*Autogenic Therapy,* New York, NY: Grune & Stratton.
4. To download a copy of the Institute of Medicine (IOM) report, go to: www.iom.edu/reports/2011/relieving-pain-in-america-a-blueprint-for-transforming-prevention-care-education-research.aspx

Index

ABOUT THE AUTHOR

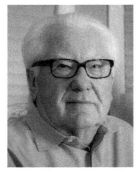

DR. KERN A. OLSON earned his doctorate from the University of Wyoming. His Internship was at the University of Oregon Medical School, Department of Medical Psychology. He continued his studies in the area of biofeedback at the Professional School of Biofeedback in San Francisco, California, and at the Albert Einstein College of Medicine in New York City. At the University of Texas, Dr. Olson studied neuropsychology assessment.

Dr. Olson has worked as a Staff Psychologist of Mental Health Programs, in private practice, as Director of Behavioral Medicine and Psychological Services, and as a psychologist in a Pain Management Center. He is a member of the American Psychological Association, the Association for Advancement of Behavior Therapy, Society of Behavioral Medicine, and the Association for Applied Psychophysiology and Biofeedback. Specific societies associated with the research of pain of which Dr. Olson is a member of are the American Pain Society, Western Pain Society, International Association for the Study of Pain, Neuromodulation Society, and Portland Pain Interest Study Group.

As a well-known pain management expert, Dr. Olson has an active history of invited lectureships and has contributed to numerous journal publications. At the time of the publication of his book, *It Hurts*, he sits on the editorial board of *Practical Pain Management* magazine and maintains a private practice in Portland, Oregon.

WELLBRIDGE BOOKS

Our focus at WellBridge Books is personal transformation, attaining health and vitality, and increasing a sense of well-being through thoughtfully written self-help books by authors who have experience and background in specialized fields of treating the whole person. Each book published by WellBridge Books is carefully selected for its ability to guide the reader in a measurable, step-wise process of self-awareness that enhances the mind, body and spirit. Whether written by a practicing or retired psychologist, counselor, medical professional, certified life coach or a certified personal trainer, each book is written in straightforward, down-to-earth language and includes creative, solution-oriented programs (often with worksheets) which provide the opportunity to build life-long bridges to lasting, healthy choices.

An imprint of Six Degrees Publishing Group, WellBridge Books is a publisher that maintains the values of our mission of "publishing extraordinary works that uplift the human spirit."

Learn more and visit our author pages at:

WellBridgeBooks.com